THE FIBROMYALGIA STORY

THE
FIBROMYALGIA
STORY

MEDICAL

AUTHORITY AND

WOMEN'S WORLDS

OF PAIN

Kristin K. Barker

 Temple University Press
PHILADELPHIA

Temple University Press
1601 North Broad Street
Philadelphia PA 19122
www.temple.edu/tempress

Library of Congress Cataloging-in-Publication Data

Barker, Kristin Kay.
   The fibromyalgia story : medical authority and women's worlds of pain / Kristin K.
Barker.
      p. cm.
   Includes bibliographical references and index.
   ISBN 1-59213-160-3 (alk. paper) – ISBN 1-59213-161-1 (pbk : alk. paper)
   1. Fibromyalgia.   I. Title.

RC927.3.B365   2005
616.7'42—dc22

                                                        2004062558

2 4 6 8 9 7 5 3 1

Contents

Acknowledgments

This book is principally about the experiences of women in pain and so it is fitting that I begin by acknowledging the women who graciously shared their experiences with me. I hope they understand that I am not suggesting that fibromyalgia is something less than a clear-cut and fully legitimate biomedical entity, but, indeed, something much more.

I would like to thank many colleagues for their intellectual input and personal support that directly and indirectly made this book possible. The faculty in the Sociology and Anthropology Department at Linfield College provided me with a rare, intellectually curious, and genuinely interdisciplinary environment in which to explore and formulate this project at its earliest stages. I am sincerely thankful to each of them. Without the hard work and dedication of the librarians at Linfield College, especially that of Frances Rasmussen in inter-library loan, this project would have been impossible. My new colleagues in the Sociology Department at Oregon State University have been supportive of my work and generous with their praise and feedback. Special thanks go to Department Chairperson Rebecca Warner for keeping her watchful (but kindly) eye on the progress of this book. Sociology colleagues outside my home institutions, especially Raka Ray and Paula Lantz, listened to me recite pieces of my argument over and over, and yet each time they helped me further clarify and focus my claims. Natalie Boero, first, as my undergraduate student and now as a medical sociologist in her own right, not only helped conduct several interviews for this study, but also proved an invaluable sounding board for working through ideas and preventing me from taking false turns at various junctures along the way.

Although I will not mention them by name, I would like to thank the fibromyalgia medical experts who agreed to answer my technical questions, face-to-face, over the phone, and via e-mail. I greatly appreciate their patience with my academician's naiveté on certain medical matters. Likewise, I would like to thank the American College of Rheumatology and the Oregon Chapter of the Arthritis Foundation for answering the many pestering questions I directed their way when I first started this research.

Special thanks also go to Peter Wissoker at Temple University Press who has been calm and helpful from the very beginning of this project. I am thankful too for the thoughtful feedback from anonymous reviewers of this manuscript who worked with others at Temple University Press. Their comments have dramatically improved the final product.

By far my greatest debt is to Val Burris. The intellectual, practical, and personal support and devotion he has bestowed on me and this project are vast. Further words about the nature and significance of his support would be cliché.

THE FIBROMYALGIA STORY

Introduction

Alice's Nightmare

lice is a single, white woman in her late forties. Approximately ten years ago she was in an accident in which her car was totaled. Doctors reported that she was lucky to have escaped with only bumps and bruises, but Alice felt as though every bone in her entire body was broken. Moreover, the intense pain would not go away. Concurrent with her peculiar pain and delayed recovery, Alice had become the primary caregiver of her mother, who had been diagnosed with a terminal illness. For several agonizing months Alice watched over her dying mother. The day after her mother's funeral Alice had hip surgery, hoping that it might lessen the pain that had persisted in the wake of her accident. The surgery failed to provide relief and, instead, it further weakened her body and amplified her symptoms.

> **Alice:** I just never recovered from the surgery. Even though I took six weeks off work, I just never recovered. I started getting lots of funny aches and pains. I would wake up in the morning and my whole arm was sore. Three or four days later that would go away and then I would get some other pain someplace else. It just kept progressing.

Alice experienced a host of new symptoms, including fatigue, blackouts, diarrhea, and migraines. Thinking that she was just run down and in need of rest, Alice spent nearly all her time in bed. No amount of sleep could offset her feeling of total exhaustion and eventually the symptoms became overwhelming. Even the simple task of lifting her arms became impossible and Alice was forced to give

1

up her twenty-year career as a beautician. Shortly thereafter, she moved in with family members who were willing to help her during a difficult time. In only a few short months, Alice had lost her physical mobility, her mother, her career, and her independence.

In the meantime, she went from doctor to doctor, but none of them could find an explanation for her symptoms. She had numerous blood tests and x-ray examinations, but findings from all the tests were normal. Before long, the doctors began to suggest that Alice's symptoms were psychosomatic.

> **Alice:** I would be hurting so bad, but all the tests were normal. By this time the doctors were starting to feel that it was all psychological. You know, the stress of the accident, the stress of mother's death, the stress of the hip surgery.

Even Alice began to question herself. She could not reconcile the discrepancy between how badly she felt and the doctors' inability to find anything wrong. Maybe she was doing this to herself, but why? It did not make sense.

> **Alice:** Why would I do this to myself? Nobody wants to be sick. Here they were telling me nothing is wrong, but I knew something was wrong. I knew this was something going on in my body.

In the absence of a compelling explanation for her intense and disabling symptoms, Alice became severely depressed and attempted to take her own life. Then, after seven years of on-going pain, depression, and countless medical examinations and diagnostic workups, her condition was diagnosed as fibromyalgia, a disorder she had never heard of. Even though her doctor told her there was no effective treatment for the condition, Alice felt a tremendous sense of relief.

> **Alice:** It was such a relief to have a name. It wasn't like anything can be done about it but finally I could say "okay, I am not crazy." It didn't really change how the doctor treated the symptoms, but I had a name. That validated it. It had a name; it was a real live thing.

Indeed, the doctors have been able to do very little for Alice in the seven years since her condition was diagnosed. Living very modestly on Social Security disability benefits, she battles severe pain and depression every day. Nevertheless, she has an occasional good day when she can get up and do something for a few hours; but then there are bad days when she drags herself out of bed only to sit and rest for hours on end. A bad day with fibromyalgia, Alice says, cannot really be called living at all; it is "just existing."

In many ways, Alice's story is emblematic of those diagnosed with the chronic pain disorder fibromyalgia. Like Alice, most who suffer from fibromyalgia are white women between the ages of thirty and fifty (Wolfe et al. 1995). As with others who have fibromyalgia, Alice describes the interplay of physical and emotional suffering in ways not easily captured by our cultural categories that tend to frame them as distinct. Also illustrative, Alice catalogs a vast collection of distressing symptoms that build to a breaking point and a corresponding sequence of painful limitations and losses. Her long and desperate search for a reason for her distress and, in its absence, the emergence of overwhelming self-doubt, is likewise typical, as is her feeling of immense relief when her suffering is at last given a name. Finally, the relentlessness of living with a debilitating, chronic illness and trying to eke out something more than just an existence during periods of relative well-being are also characteristic of those living with fibromyalgia. Because Alice's experience is like that of many of those who suffer from fibromyalgia, her story is an appropriate place to begin. Moreover, by keeping her story close at hand, this inquiry will not lose sight of the human suffering that typifies fibromyalgia.

Fibromyalgia Syndrome: Some Basics

Fibromyalgia, strictly speaking, is not a disease. Rather, it is a clinical "syndrome" represented by a collection of symptoms, such as chronic, widespread pain and a host of associated symptoms, including fatigue, headaches, sleep irregularities, irritable bowel syndrome, irritable bladder syndrome, cognitive and mood disorders, and increased sensitivity to stimuli, to name just a few. In fact, partly tongue-in-cheek, the best-selling fibromyalgia syndrome (FMS) self-help book refers to the condition as "Irritable Everything Syndrome" (Starlanyl and Copeland 1996: 13).[1]

Fibromyalgia syndrome is both common and debilitating. Although determining the actual prevalence and incidence of FMS is impossible to do with precision, it is estimated that between 2 and 5 percent of the general population meet the FMS criteria, with significantly higher rates for women than men (Gran 2003; Neumann and Buskila 2003; White et al. 1999; Wolfe et al. 1995). The numbers are dramatic: during the last several decades more than six million Americans have been diagnosed with FMS (Abeles 1998; Goldenberg 1999). For millions of sufferers, the consequences of FMS symptoms are often devastating: studies demonstrate significantly compromised functional ability, health status, and quality of life, with little long-term improvement in well-being over time (Goldenberg 2002; Henriksson and Burckhardt 1996; Wolfe et al. 1997a). The costs in human suffering associated with such a common and disabling disorder are staggering, and the financial costs related to direct health care expenditures and public and private disability claims are increasingly burdensome (Osterweis et al. 1987; Wolfe et al. 1997b).

Fibromyalgia syndrome is also controversial. The most straightforward explanation for the sudden and dramatic rise of FMS would be that the tools of medicine have only recently discovered or revealed what has historically eluded the medical gaze or had been crudely captured in accounts of "vapors," "nerves," "hysteria," or "neurasthenia." However, such a scientifically deterministic account of the emergence of FMS is impossible to sustain. Medical science has yet to make FMS visible. Although patients experience intense muscular pain, no muscle or joint deterioration can be seen through imaging techniques such as x-ray films, magnetic resonance imaging (MRI), or computed axial tomography (CAT) scans. Likewise, blood tests also fail to reveal abnormalities. A growing body of medical research points to potential organic abnormalities but no objective marker of FMS currently exists; it evades our modern laboratory arsenal. Consequently, as with chronic fatigue syndrome (CFS), which is identified by most patients, physicians, and researchers as either the same or a sister disorder, FMS remains a contested illness.

Nevertheless, rheumatologists, the medical specialists most closely affiliated with FMS, established formal diagnostic criteria for FMS in 1990, based on their findings from an extensive sixteen-center panel study. The American College of Rheumatology (ACR) criteria for FMS include the subjective report of widespread pain for at least three months and pain in at least eleven of eighteen "tender points." Patients must report mild or greater tenderness when these points are pressed firmly during a medial examination. The diagnostic tender point locations are seen in the medical illustration of The Three Graces from the ACR's criteria study published in *Arthritis and Rheumatism* (Figure 1).

After the physician eliminates the possibility that a patient's pain results from known organic causes (e.g., cancer or multiple sclerosis), a tender point examination can be performed to confirm the FMS diagnosis. Although the ACR criteria are still used for research purposes, in clinical practice the formal criteria are not strictly upheld. In 1992, a working panel of FMS experts recommended that an individual with fewer than the eleven required tender points may still have a diagnosis of FMS if he or she experiences several of the associated symptoms that cluster together as part of the wider syndrome (Csillag 1992).

In sum, the indicators of FMS are determined subjectively, by exclusion, and inexactly. Physicians' laying their hands on patients and eliciting and interpreting a patient's self-report is truly anachronistic in an era of high-tech biomedicine. As Paul Starr (1982) reminds us, the rise of modern medical authority is principally the outcome of scientific instrumentation

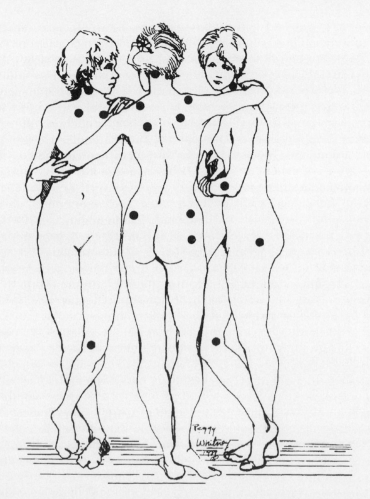

Figure 1 Fibromyalgia Tender Points. Frederick Wolfe, Hugh Smythe, Muhammed Yunus, Robert Bennett, Claire Bombardier, Don Goldenberg, Peter Tugwell, Stephen Campbell, Mich Abeles, Patricia Clark, Robert Gatter, Daniel Hamaty, James Lessard, Alan Lichtbrown, Alfonse Masi, Glenn McCain, W. John Reynolds, Thomas Romano, I. John Russell, and Robert Sheon. "The Amerian College of Rheumatology 1990 criteria for the classification of fibromyalgia." *Arthritis and Rheumatism*, copyright 1990. Reprinted by permission of Wiley-Liss, Inc., a subsidiary of John Wiley & Sons, Inc.

that made disease within the body visible to physicians, thereby reducing their reliance on a patient's subjective evaluation. Likewise, Michel Foucault (1975) argues that medicine derives its power from its penetrating *gaze* into the body, allowing it to see and know the body in a way not visible or knowable to the patient himself or herself. Because medical authority is premised on the ability to make patients' subjective symptoms objectively and precisely visible, the FMS diagnosis is medically precarious.

The elusiveness of FMS is amplified by the fact that no clear explanations exist for what causes the disorder. In some cases, FMS symptoms appear in the wake of viral illness or physical or emotional trauma; in many cases, however, the symptoms materialize unexplainably. There are competing hypotheses about the underlying pathogenesis of the disorder, but they remain speculative and provisional. Further confounding is the fact there are no effective treatments for the condition. Patients are treated with a host of general drug and behavioral therapies (e.g., analgesics, anti-inflammatories, antidepressants, physical exercise, relaxation techniques), but clinical trials have been limited and show only minimal and inconsistent recompense (Goldenberg 1999; Redondo et al. 2004).

Given the inability of medicine to read FMS objectively from the body—together with its ill-specified pathogenesis and treatment—it is not surprising that there is no uniform answer to the question: "Is FMS *real* or not?" The question itself is ripe with cultural assumptions that deeply inform the institution of medicine. Clinician researchers, for all intents and purposes, are divided between those who believe that FMS is a disorder with some underlying organic component and those who do not. Even though the limits of such an overly simplistic divide are generally recognized, it is along this fault line that the FMS wars are currently being waged. In a recent editorial exchange in the *Journal of Rheumatology*, rheumatolgists fiercely attacked one another in the latest round in the ongoing FMS debate. First came a series of hard-hitting editorials asserting that the diagnosis should be abandoned on grounds it lacks scientific justification and encourages distressed individuals toward exaggerated illness behavior (Ehrlich 2003; Wolfe 2003). Then came the counterattack. Advocates of the diagnosis chronicled clinical studies suggestive of biophysical abnormalities associated with FMS and heralded a time in the very near future when the evidence supporting the existence of the disorder would be so overwhelming as to silence "even the most violent FM-beaters" (White 2004: 636). Although both sides insist the debate is more or less over and their respective side has won, the existence of this recently published dispute makes clear that the scientific facts about FMS remain hotly contested.

All of this medical uncertainty stands in sharp contrast to the subjective experience of the syndrome. As illustrated in the case of Alice, the accounts of those suffering from FMS are strikingly vivid and highly compelling. In most cases, the intense pain, fatigue, and other distressing symptoms are experienced as debilitating, with social, family, and work life seriously compromised and sometimes destroyed. This experience is juxtaposed to years, sometimes decades, of seeking a medical explanation and being told by physician after physician that "nothing is wrong." Consequently, like Alice, those who suffer from FMS find themselves in an epistemological purgatory in which they must reconcile the deeply felt contradiction between their subjective certainty of their symptoms and the inability of medical science to demonstrate their objective existence. This epistemological purgatory erodes the self and creates a context in which having the condition diagnosed by a physician who believes in the disorder is transformative. A diagnosis after years of unexplainable suffering bestows validation and legitimization, as well as a sense of coherence and order, to a vast collection of confusing and disabling symptoms.

The FMS Story

This book is about the coming together of women patients, like Alice, with a host of distressing symptoms, and a small cadre of rheumatologists—referred to here as diagnostic entrepreneurs. It describes how the collaboration between women patients and rheumatologists resulted in the creation of "fibromyalgia syndrome." To claim that fibromyalgia is the outcome of this collaboration is not dismissive of the real suffering of those with this diagnosis, nor is it an accusation of medical malfeasance. Rather, the intent is to draw attention to how rheumatologists organized, understood, and labeled women's suffering through specific medical practices and how and why this conceptual framework compellingly intersected with women's experience and understanding of their own distress. The creation of FMS, as will be demonstrated, is indeed a predictable outcome, pushed by tendencies within both medicine and the social and cultural terrain in which medicine is practiced and consumed.

The FMS debate is highly polemical. For many who suffer from FMS, the world is divided into the "fibro friendly"—those who believe that FMS is a "real" physical disease—and a vast array of enemies who raise misgivings about the diagnosis or suggest that nonbiological factors (i.e., emotions or mental status) play a dominant role in the condition. As noted above, the debate within the medical community is no less polarized and divisive. In the context of such conflict, it will no doubt disappoint and frustrate many readers that I do not take a side (in particular, *their* side) in the FMS debate in the pages that follow. This stance, however, is not simply one of waffling or straddling opposing positions. My goal is not to reveal the "truth" about FMS, but to articulate an alternative position that moves us beyond the current framework within which the search for the meaning of FMS has taken place and to transcend the current impasse in the FMS debate. More specifically, my aim is to describe the *social processes* and *social conditions* that interact to promote the organization of certain experiences into FMS, both as a category of biomedical knowledge and as a subjective framework of meaning and identity. Thus, the question to be addressed is not whether FMS is real or "all in their heads," but rather *why* and *how* FMS functions as a framework that gives meaning to experience. This book, in short, is principally about the *idea* of FMS.

Data for this study include twenty-five years of FMS research publications indexed in *MEDLINE*, interviews with thirty women diagnosed with FMS, and selected FMS self-help materials. Some gaps have been filled with information gathered from other sources. These include interviews with four men diagnosed with FMS, five nationally recognized FMS researchers, several additional interviews with staff from state or national FMS-related organizations, and my observations from dozens of FMS workshops, conferences, and support group meetings across two states over a period of several years. In all cases, details have been omitted or changed to protect identities.

Sociology of Knowledge and the Social Construction of Illness

From its inception as a discipline, sociology has approached ideas as reflections of the specific historical and social environments in which they are produced. In different ways, the founding sociological thinkers—Karl Marx (1818–1883), Max Weber (1864–1920), and Emile Durkheim (1858–1917)—each addressed the relationship between the ideas or beliefs of a society and the social and material conditions of that society. In his book, *Ideology and Utopia,* Karl Mannheim (1936) codified this general stance by directing sociology to study empirically the "relationalism" of people's ideas, by which he meant to study how people's ideas are conditioned by historical context as well as their station in society. More contemporarily, feminist and postmodern sociologists have showcased the link between our ideas and our social locations in race, class, and gender hierarchies of power (Collins 1991; Smith 1987). This venerable tradition—often called the "sociology of knowledge"—studies ideas not as expressions of *truth* per se, but as the realized expression of particular social interests within particular social systems and contexts (Merton 1973). In other words, from a sociology of knowledge perspective, ideas are social *constructions* (Berger and Luckmann 1967).

Sociologists study the social construction of many different ideas, but some researchers are explicitly interested in studying ideas about illness. Such a perspective emphasizes the relationship between ideas about illness and the expression, perception, understanding, and response to illness at both the individual and societal level (Conrad and Schneider 1992; Foucault 1975; Freidson 1971; Illich 1976). Historical and cross-cultural comparisons are effective ways to illustrate the social constructionist claim. Imagine, for example, two societies: one that defines illness principally as the outcome of moral failings or spiritual transgressions (on the part of individuals or communities) and another that defines illness principally as the result of organic disturbance within an individual human body. Who (or even what) is identified as "ill" in these two societies will differ dramatically, as will arrangements for how and by whom illness is to be treated. In addition, the subjective experience and meaning of being ill will be markedly dissimilar because the two societies provide very different interpretive frameworks of the illness experience. In one society, "the shamed" stand before the shaman or priest who rights the wrong, cleanses the soul, or grants mercy; in the other, the individual victim of disease—"the patient"—seeks the physician's technical skills to restore or fix his or her wounded body.

In a related fashion, social constructionists explore why particular illnesses exist in one place and not another, or appear and then quickly disappear in the very same place. In many societies, for example, women do not experience premenstrual syndrome (PMS) or anorexia nervosa, whereas the turn-of-century epidemics of hysteria and neurasthenia in Western societies have now largely faded from view. These examples effectively advance the social constructionist claim that illness and disease are more than fixed physical realities; they are phenomena shaped by social experiences, shared cultural traditions, and shifting frameworks of knowledge.

From a social constructionist perspective, the task is not necessarily to determine which of the above two societies has the *correct* ideas about illness or which of illnesses found only in certain places or certain times are actually *real*. Instead, the task is to determine how and why particular ideas about illness appear, change, or persist for reasons that are partly independent of their validity. For example, close attention is paid to how and why particular definitions or ideas about illness became dominant in particular places and times and how they marginalize or silence alternative ideas (Conrad and Schneider 1992; Starr 1982; Tesh 1988). Additional questions follow: What factors help explain why one society defines illness in moral terms, whereas another eschews such ideas in favor of observable anatomic abnormality? What are the central consequences—for the society at large and for afflicted individuals—of one set of ideas versus another? What dynamics are at play in the appearance and disappearance of a certain illness or in the existence of an illness in one place but its absence elsewhere?

Although these are some archetypal social constructionist questions, questions about reality and truth inevitably percolate to the surface. Do not some ideas about illness simply better reflect the reality and truth about illness? Does not the scientific disease model explain and treat illness better than a religious approach? Are the above examples of illnesses that are culture-bound or historically short-lived real illnesses? Do objective illnesses not exist? Does not death prove that illness is not a social construction?

Not everyone agrees what calling an illness "socially constructed" implies about its real existence (or lack thereof). As used in this study, a social constructionist position does *not* imply that our illnesses have no objective basis whatsoever, nor does saying that an illness is socially constructed deny its possible biophysical reality (Brown 1995; Freidson 1971).[2] To show that our ideas are socially and historically determined does not imply, in and of themselves, that they are deeply distorted or false. In effect, there are two levels of inquiry and these levels can be kept separate: one can accept the empirical evidence that our ideas are socially constructed without drawing the conclusion that they are, for that reason, necessarily false (Mannheim 1936: 267).[3] In short, social constructionism need not dispense with the notion of reality, although reality, as such, is not its central focus (Berger and Luckmann 1967). We will return to these claims later in the book, but for now it is sufficient to observe that our ideas about illness can be specific to a time and place, contingent on particular social interests rather than others, consequential in particular and noninherent ways, and *also*, in full or in part, empirically valid. In brief, an illness, in principle, can be both real *and* socially constructed (Hacking 1999).[4]

Cultural Hegemony of Biomedical Knowledge

In our advanced capitalist society, it is difficult to overstate the influence of *biomedicine* in shaping our ideas about illness and the body. Biomedicine is a term that captures the nature of important changes that emerged in Western medical practice between the late 1800s and early 1900s. This period marked the coming together of medicine and the laboratory-based biological sciences (Shryock 1974; Warner 1986). Medicine's reliance on knowledge of biological processes and its production of knowledge charting these processes have marked a significant transformation in medical practice. Even as the practice of medicine at the dawn of the twenty-first century differs greatly from that of a century ago, the term "biomedicine" represents the historical thread that unites the practice of medicine in two otherwise different eras. In brief, biomedicine is medical practice based on the principles, methods, and technologies of the biological life sciences, and it has tremendous cultural authority in matters of illness.

For example, biomedicine alone is the final arbitrator in determining the existence of a disease. A disease does not exist, so to speak, until the social institution of biomedicine creates a representative diagnostic category. Oftentimes, the creation of a new biomedical diagnosis represents a scientific breakthrough or set of breakthroughs. New biological pathologies are discovered that account for a particular human distress and we rightly see an expansion of biomedical authority over that particular human experience. In other cases, however, no straightforward scientific justification exists for how and why a particular human experience comes to be organized and represented under a biomedical diagnosis. These latter, less straightforward, cases are of greatest interest to sociologists (Brown 1995). In particular, sociologists maintain that the "politics of interpretation" are at play when certain aspects of human life come to be framed medically in the absence of unambiguous medical triumphs (Conrad and Schneider 1992).

Largely in recognition that biomedicine can garner authority in the absence of clear scientific justification, the social constructionist perspective often goes hand in hand with the concept of *medicalization*. Medicalization refers to the processes by which human experiences that are neither inherently nor fully medical in character come to be identified as essentially medical in nature. Often this includes the medicalization of social and personal problems: for example, the medicalization of social deviance (Conrad and Schneider 1992). Calling the *drunk* an *alcoholic* simultaneously captures the medicalization of both a social and a personal problem. In other instances, it is appropriate to speak of the medicalization of life itself. Such is the case with the medicalization of natural physical changes, ranging from the profound (e.g., senility) to the trivial (e.g., male pattern baldness). Through medicalization, normal complaints become medical conditions, often with significant consequences.

Medicalization, for example, can obscure the *social* forces that influence our health and well-being. One of the central assumptions of the biomedical model is that disease is the result of specific bodily dysfunction. Insofar as disease is defined as biological states residing within the human body, the relationship between social ills and ill health can be distorted or overlooked. This is seen clearly in the recent trend toward "biologizing" depression. As the dominant story becomes one about the link between mood and a genetic predisposition toward neurochemical alternations, we stop telling other stories, such as those that include details about the association between despair and the social environment (Kaplan 2000: 134). Medicalization can also grant the institution of medicine undue authority over our bodies and lives, thereby limiting individual autonomy and functioning as a form of social control. As Ivan Illich (1976: 6) warned more than a quarter century ago: "[s]ociety has transferred to physicians the exclusive right to determine what constitutes sickness, who is or might become sick, and what shall be done to such people." Since Illich's writing, however, we have come to understand that medicalization rarely is exclusively the result of the medical profession's imperialistic claims over our bodies and lives. As patients, we sometimes actively participate in or demand the medicalization of our experiences as we earnestly seek meaning for our suffering. Both impulses toward medicalization—professional expansion and patient demand—make sense in a context where biomedicine has tremendous cultural authority.

In fact, these two impulses present different paths toward medicalization that roughly correspond to important changes in biomedicine between the early and the latter part of the twentieth century. One of the many unmistakable changes witnessed during biomedicine's century-long reign is its increasingly omnipresent character. Whereas early modern biomedicine was a separate social-institutional field into which *patients* where pushed, pulled, or otherwise wandered from time to time for discrete treatment, today biomedicine is also an elaborate and vast set of diffuse practices, beliefs, and products that continually permeate the self and everyday life. For example, we are routinely exposed to health-related information, services, and identities—an immense web of commodities and discourses that cross most social–institutional boundaries and are neither exclusively produced nor controlled by medical professionals (Clarke et al. 2003).[5] No longer contained within traditional clinic walls or professional and expert institutions, biomedicine seeps into and grows out of our everyday world, giving rise to new types of knowledge, consumer practices, patient movements, and socially constructed identities. Fueled by capitalism's hyperevolved consumer culture, one might say that the ubiquitous character of contemporary biomedicine facilitates a spirit of "do-it-yourself" medicalization.

Drawing on social constructionist tenets, feminist scholars have demonstrated how women's bodies and experiences have been particularly susceptible to medicalization. The reasons for this tendency are complex, but at the center of feminist thinking on the topic is the ancient Western intellectual assumption, well entrenched within biomedical thought, that equates masculine with universality and feminine with particularity. From Aristotle to the birth of modern biomedicine, the male body stands for the essential or normalized body. Given that male physiology is defined as normative, female physiology is necessarily an aberration. In other words, borrowing Simone de Beauvoir's (1989) central insight, men and men's bodies represent the biomedical standard and women and women's bodies are the biomedical "other." It is but a short step to define as abnormal what are indeed normal aspects of women's embodiment. For example, women's natural reproductive functions are routinely medicalized (e.g., pregnancy, childbirth, menstruation, menopause) or are considered likely causative culprits in female maladies (e.g., hysteria comes from *hystera*, the Greek word for womb) (Ehrenreich and English 1973; Martin 1987). Not only does this orientation beget the medicalization of women's routine lives, it can also bias and misdirect biomedical research and practice in relation to women's health.[6] That being said, women have themselves been very proactive in processes of medicalization—perhaps, as it has been argued, because it represents one of a few avenues afforded them to pursue their needs and gain access to resources in a society characterized by gender inequality (Lorber 1997; Riessman 1983; Theriot 1983).

The themes raised by a social constructionist perspective, including the dominant and increasingly ubiquitous role that biomedicine plays in defining and organizing our complaints into disease (and syndrome) categories and the corresponding tendencies toward medicalization, generally, and of women's experiences, particularly, apply to the case at hand—namely, the social construction of FMS.

Social Construction of FMS: An Overview

The next two chapters address the social construction of FMS as a category of biomedical knowledge, based on an analysis of twenty-five years of published FMS medical research and commentary. Chapter 1 provides a detailed summary of how a group of rheumatologists developed the idea of FMS and the subsequent knowledge claims and counterclaims that have developed about that idea over time. The FMS story begins with and continues to be shaped by rheumatology's professional ambitions, as well as its setbacks, vis-à-vis its attempts to translate common and elusive symptoms into a coherent medical diagnosis. Chapter 2 retells this story, but builds on research into women's health to make the case that FMS represents a highly feminized mode of distress. The principal argument to emerge from Chapter 2 is that much of women's somatic distress is readily medicalized as FMS; yet, at the same time, standard biomedical practice and nomenclature obscure the very fact that the diagnosis is a template expressly for *women's* distress. Beyond the specific case of FMS, Chapters 1 and 2 point to the broader incompatibility between the character of women's somatic suffering and the practices of biomedicine—the consequences of which include the feminization of a long lineage of past and present contested diagnoses. Readers who are not interested in the technical details of how rheumatolgists created the diagnostic criteria for FMS and how other clinician researchers continue to grapple with this construction can skip Chapters 1 and 2.

Although the story of FMS would never have been written but for the entrepreneurial efforts of rheumatologists described in Chapters 1 and 2, in some ways, the heart (or at least the soul) of this book begins with Chapter 3. Based on interviews with thirty women with conditions diagnosed as FMS, Chapters 3 through 8 address the relationship between the idea of FMS as a category of biomedical knowledge and the subsequent experience of those who suffer from FMS. Chapter 3 introduces the illness experience literature and outlines how illness narratives provide an empirical tool for understanding human suffering unlike the tools used in biomedicine. For example, although there is a lack of conceptual coherence to FMS from a biomedical perspective—that is, not all who suffer from FMS become sick in the same way or have the same set of symptoms—a shared resonance is found in the narrative accounts of those living with FMS. Chapters 4 through 7 describe those narrative similarities. More specifically, Chapter 4 presents a detailed account of FMS symptoms and how the experience of those symptoms erodes the self and all that is taken for granted. The focus of Chapter 5 is how the prolonged and frustrating search for symptom meaning that characterizes the FMS experience becomes infused with a gender ideology that presupposes women's irrationality, leaving those who suffer feeling both bewildered and discredited. The stage is thus set for Chapter 6, which describes how, after a long period of invalidation, women patients are transformed by and embrace the diagnosis of FMS, even as they face the limitations of living with a contested illness. The collective nature of the search for illness coherence and selfhood is the topic of Chapter 7, which examines the role of the FMS self-help community in reaffirming the "realness" of FMS, validating sufferers' subjective experience in the face of lay and medical skepticism, and aiding in the formation of a new identity based on the shared experience of being diagnosed with FMS. Chapter 8 provides an analysis of the available social epidemiology of FMS in an effort to bring the central claims of this book into sharper focus, namely, that FMS is both a socially constructed category of biomedical knowledge and a cognitive structure that gives meaning to women's worlds of pain.

But, the reader must be reminded that this is not a study about the biomedical reality of FMS. Such investigations are best left to biomedical researchers. This is a sociological study about the idea of FMS as a biomedical concept created and studied by clinicians and then applied to and used by lay people. One could denote this epistemological stance by using "FMS" in quotes throughout this book; to avoid stylistic awkwardness, such an approach is not used. Nevertheless, the reader needs to remain mindful that the when sociologists study "reality" they are "[l]ogically, if not stylistically... stuck with the quotation marks" (Berger and Luckmann 1967: 2).

1

The Diagnostic Making of Fibromyalgia Syndrome

ccording to Robert Bennett, one of the national figures in fibromyalgia syndrome (FMS) research and treatment, fibromyalgia is a descriptive "construct developed by rheumatologists to account for a common group of patients that they see in their routine practice" (Bennett 1999a: 1). Although FMS originated as an intellectual construct developed by rheumatologists to help in the study and treatment of a common group of patients, the idea of FMS has since become reified at the level of both knowledge and experience. Much of this book is devoted to describing the phenomenon of FMS at the experiential level. But before those who suffer could come to organize their experiences around the diagnosis of FMS, the diagnosis itself had to be made and formalized as biomedical knowledge. This chapter describes how rheumatologists developed the construct or idea of FMS and the subsequent debate about that idea within the institutional field of biomedicine, generally, and the subspecialty of rheumatology, in particular.

The Subspecialty of Rheumatology

Rheumatology has been, and continues to be, the field of medicine most closely associated with FMS. Rheumatology is a subfield of internal medicine and, in general terms, its claim of professional expertise involves conditions of the musculoskeletal system. Although current biomedical science rejects the premise that FMS is a musculoskeletal disorder, those who suffer from it experience intense muscle and joint pain, which places rheumatologists at the center of the FMS story.

Rheumatology as a field of American medicine emerged between the 1920s and 1940s (Kersley and Glyn 1991; Smyth et al. 1985). Following the lead of efforts underway in Europe, Dr. Ralph Pemberton was the first American physician to call himself a rheumatologist and limit his practice to rheumatic disease. In 1926, Pemberton opened the first arthritis clinic in the United States at Pennsylvania's Presbyterian Hospital in Philadelphia. At roughly the same time, several prestigious medical schools, including Harvard and Columbia, initiated academic departments of rheumatology, bringing attention and respectability to the enterprise through their residency training. Paralleling these practical and educational ventures were efforts to create a professional organization. In 1927, the American Committee for the Control of Rheumatism was formed, which ten years later changed its name to the American Rheumatism Association (and would later still change its name to the American College of Rheumatology). During the 1940s, as its membership grew, the America Rheumatism Association (ARA) began to have a discernible professional impact. For example, a dramatic indication of professional consolidation occurred in 1941, when the ARA developed and adopted the first classification for rheumatic diseases. In 1947, the American Rheumatism Foundation (now called the Arthritis Foundation) was created in partnership with the ARA to provide research funds to clinician researchers, enticing a new generation into the field. By the end of the 1940s, a nascent field of rheumatology was well underway.

In contrast to the steady progress in the organizational development of rheumatology between the mid 1920s and 1950, there was little corresponding success in the treatment of most rheumatic diseases. Between 1880 and 1950, the curative promise of medicine was found in the field of bacteriology. As such, rheumatic disorders were primarily treated as though infectious in origin. This approach did not result in many successes, although a few exceptions existed, including the elimination of arthritic conditions caused by gonorrhea, syphilis, and tuberculosis. Additionally, observations linking hemolytic streptococci and rheumatic fever among soldiers in WWII led to the near total elimination of this disease in the United States (Smyth et al. 1985). Overall, however, the developing field of rheumatology had little to boast of in terms of its general therapeutic efficacy until the end of the 1940s.

In 1949, researchers discovered the therapeutic benefits of cortisone for the treatment of arthritis. Even taking into consideration the negative side effects of cortisone and its synthetic siblings, this development represents the zenith of rheumatology's therapeutic promise. The introduction of corticosteroids to treat rheumatic inflammation is such a significant benchmark in the development of rheumatology that many divide the field's history in terms of "BC" and "AC" (*before cortisone* and *after cortisone*) (Kersley and Glyn 1991: 84). The therapeutic euphoria in the immediate AC period facilitated the establishment of the Institute of Arthritis and Metabolic Disease within the National Institute of Health in 1950. Along with Arthritis Foundation monies, research funds from the Institute added considerably to rheumatology's professional potential and allure.

During the next several decades, there were other significant signs of rheumatology's institutionalization as a specialty in American medicine. In 1958, for example, the ARA established its official journal *Arthritis and Rheumatism*, thereby creating a specialty-based forum for peer-reviewed scientific exchange. This journal remains the most cited rheumatology journal worldwide (Weinblatt 2002). Another watershed for rheumatology was the establishment of board certification. The first examination for certification in rheumatology was given in 1972 by the American Board of Internal Medicine, thus formalizing rheumatology as a subspecialty. In many regards, this step represented the completion of rheumatology's formal professional development. In the language of the sociology of professions, it had formally established its professional jurisdiction (Abbott 1988; Freidson 1971; Larson 1977). Rheumatology had a unique and legitimate claim of professional expertise and it created a gate-keeping mechanism to ensure that only trained and certified clinicians had legitimate access to that jurisdiction.

Rheumatology is now a small, but recognized, field in contemporary American medicine. There are approximately 4,000 board-certified rheumatolgists, many of whom are members of rheumatology's professional association, the American College of Rheumatology (ACR) (American Board of Internal Medicine 2004).[1] Yet, in many regards, the field of rheumatology remains professionally precarious. One important reason for its precariousness is that it has few clear answers or solutions for the wide range of illnesses that fall under its jurisdiction. The common conditions that bring patients to rheumatolgists—various types of arthritis, lupus, osteoporosis, and fibromyalgia—are dissimilar, chronic, and complex. In fact, many of the disorders that fall to rheumatology are not musculoskeletal disorders at all, despite the fact that the rheumatology's professional expertise involves the musculoskeletal system. Accordingly, rheumatology has no overarching conceptual paradigms or unified principles to organize intellectually the illnesses and treatments of its routine sphere of authority. It is not inaccurate to say that most rheumatological diseases continue to be poorly understood and poorly managed.[2]

For example, rheumatology's contemporary therapeutic repertoire includes a collection of unsatisfactory options. In addition to a host of newer steroidal drugs, countless nonsteroidal anti-inflammatory drugs (NSAID) are now available. The sheer number of steroidal and NSAID options indicates that not one is fully satisfactory, either in terms of effectiveness or safety, for the treatment of rheumatic patients (Weinblatt 2002). Although current excitement exists about new disease-modifying anti-rheumatic drugs (DMARD), which through immune suppression may slow the progression of rheumatoid arthritis, they do not cure the underlying pathology and they bring a host of problematic side effects. In sum, clinical practice in rheumatology primarily involves partially managing patient's symptoms, whereas the goal of eradicating rheumatologic illnesses remains as elusive to the contemporary rheumatologists as it did to Ralph Pemberton, the father of American rheumatology, in the 1920s.

Unquestionably, the factors outlined above contribute to the current gloomy mood of the subspecialty. A palpable sense is found among its practitioners that rheumatology is facing hard times. There are still very few rheumatologists. Moreover, the number of trainees entering rheumatology programs is falling, suggesting that their numbers will only decline further. That rheumatology programs are not widely represented at academic medical centers both illustrates and perpetuates the field's failure to thrive. Additionally, the managed care environment presents ever greater threats. The cost-benefit model that characterizes the new era of health outcomes research bodes poorly for a subfield dependent on justifiable referrals when patient improvement, as a rule, is negligible in relation to the expense. Likewise, health economists have determined that rheumatology clinics do not benefit a hospital's bottom line, making its future in corporate run (and nonprofit, but corporate-like run) health care uncertain (Weinblatt 2002).

As a brief aside: Some of the struggles facing rheumatology parallel those facing other specialists and, to some degree, the medical profession as a whole. For example, today all physicians face complex, chronic illnesses that are often poorly understood or poorly managed. Likewise, rheumatology is not the only specialty whose overarching conceptual focus fails to account meaningfully for the range of conditions that fall under its purview. By contrast, the most prestigious specialty—surgery—has a very clearly defined conceptual jurisdiction.[3] Lastly, all specialties and, indeed, all medical practitioners, have felt the impact of dramatic changes in the health-care delivery system during the last several decades brought on by managed care. None of these parallels, however, belie the foregoing characterization of rheumatology as a relatively marginal professional player within the institution of medicine and a subfield marked by few glamorous theoretical or therapeutic payoffs.

In this highly condensed historical account of rheumatology, a key detail has been intentionally omitted. Whereas the subfield of rheumatology was established to study and treat disorders of the musculoskeletal system, it has come to treat patients primarily on the basis of the symptomatic experience of pain. Much has been said and written about pain's biomedical elusiveness (Scarry 1985). No objective evidence of pain exists; only a patient's subjective testimony. In this way, pain is "a medical object distinct from those that can be directly read from the body or discovered through laboratory tests" (Baszanger 1995: 8). As a result, the world of biomedicine has not treated pain as an end in and of itself (much to the regret of chronic pain sufferers), but rather as a diagnostic clue or tool (Baszanger 1995; Morris 1991). Clinicians trace pain backward, so to speak, to the true object of biomedicine: the organic condition producing the experience of pain. Such a strategic stance vis-à-vis pain can be understood, given its elusive and nonparadigmatic qualities. Biomedicine seeks a certainty that pain simply fails to surrender.

Although pain stands at the margins of biomedicine, it stands at the center of rheumatology. In effect, pain has become the conceptual justification for rheumatology. More than anything else, this fact accounts for rheumatology's imprecisely defined professional jurisdiction, relatively inglorious history marked by only modest therapeutic successes, and lack of prestige relative to many other medical specialties. The professional limitations of rheumatology, therefore, are largely a result of the profession's close association with pain, its explanation, and its treatment. For example, because pain falls within rheumatology's jurisdiction, the subfield has found itself historically and contemporarily facing a mass of patient referrals that share, with any certainty, only one thing—the subjective experience of bodily pain. In some cases, rheumatologists have been able to trace pain backward to reveal its organic foundations, but in many cases this strategic approach bears no fruit. Consequently, much of the clinical content of rheumatology is this unsorted, residual patient mass (Kersley and Glyn 1991: 79), and the attempt to create a paradigm from such a heterogeneous patient mass represents the ongoing professional challenge of rheumatology.

From the vast and disparate residual category of patients sent to rheumatologists, the diagnostic category FMS emerged and, as such, FMS illustrates rheumatology's historical relationship to, and struggle with, pain more generally. The following remarks, which appear in a special issue of *Balliere's Clinical Rheumatology* devoted to the fibromyalgia debate, illustrate the spirit of this ongoing enterprise.

> [R]heumatologists, perhaps more than other clinical specialists, have always seen pain in itself, and the associated disability, as a proper part of their remit, beyond the demands of diagnosis. The *Annals of Rheumatism* in the 1940s, for example, contain many wide-ranging descriptions of people in pain whose detailed histories related to war traumas and the psychosocial circumstances of their lives. Whether the designation of "psychogenic rheumatism" in many of these cases was helpful or not is less important than the powerful sense communicated by these case-studies, of concern for the individual's distress beyond the need for a rheumatological diagnosis (Croft and Silman 1999: xi).

But a need and demand arose for the rheumatological diagnosis of fibromyalgia and its creation must be seen as part of a central professional struggle of rheumatology: giving medical representation to individuals' subjective distress. Leading FMS expert, Don Goldenberg, explains: "Fibromyalgia is simply a label to use when patients have chronic, unexplained diffuse pain" (Goldenberg 1999: 781). Goldenberg speaks from authority, because he was among a small handful of rheumatologists who originally developed the label "fibromyalgia" and formalized it as a category of biomedical knowledge that now gives representation to the subjective suffering of millions.

The Character of Biomedical Diagnoses

Diagnosing a patient's distressing symptoms is at the heart of biomedical practice. Crucial for both physician and patient, a diagnosis represents the physician's comprehension of the patient's experience. Importantly, a diagnosis gives the physician a medical plan of action to treat or aid the patient in his or her return to health. For the patient, a diagnosis gives meaning and legitimacy to worrying symptoms and provides a framework for what he or she is facing. For all these reasons, when a patient presents distressing symptoms to a physician, both parties may find even a bad diagnosis better than no diagnosis at all (Rosenberg 1997: xviii). A diagnosis effectively legitimizes both parties and the doctor-patient relationship itself.

Medical nomenclature is the collection of diagnoses available to physicians. More than just an unorganized list of disease and disorders, nomenclature is a framework of classification that organizes and represents biomedicine's formal knowledge (Abbott 1988). For example, diseases are classified together in terms of bodily organs or systems, shared etiology, pathophysiology, and the like. Such a system of classification represents, among other things, a map of the medical profession's jurisdiction: it represents the conditions over which biomedicine has a legitimate claim of authority and expertise. Nomenclature is not a fixed system but rather a continually revised expression of biomedical knowledge. The consistent trend in nomenclature is toward an increasing number of diagnoses and classification categories (as well as subdiagnoses and subclassifications)—a trend highly apparent in the historical expansion of rheumatological nomenclature.[4]

Historian Charles Rosenberg remarks that a disease does not exist "until it is named" (Rosenberg 1997: xiii).[5] In a similar vein, sociologist Phil Brown (1995) proposes that a disease comes into existence only with the creation of a diagnostic category. Of course, neither Rosenberg nor Brown denies the material existence of disease outside of its diagnostic naming. Instead, their shared claim is that a disease does not exist *socially* until the social institution of biomedicine names it. In practice, the creation of a new diagnostic name simultaneously declares the existence of a condition and legitimizes biomedicine's professional claim of authority and expertise in relationship to that condition (Freidson 1971). The creation of a new diagnosis, and the inclusion of that diagnostic name within medical nomenclature, represent an *expansion* of biomedicine's professional jurisdiction and might, therefore, be labeled *entrepreneurial.*

The professional task of biomedicine is to determine whether the unorganized and subjective symptoms of patients can be organized and measured in terms that fall within its jurisdiction. It is through the practices and principles of diagnostic research that medicine makes (or fails to make) a new diagnostic category and, therefore, expands (or fails to expand) its jurisdiction. In particular, case-controlled clinical studies comparing individuals believed to have a condition (patients) with those lacking the condition (controls) is a dominant practice used in diagnostic research. This is a simple and familiar research design. A disorder's existence depends on whether it can be translated into biomedical *markers* present among the patients but absent among the controls. The marker or combination of markers with the best balance of sensitivity (the ability to select those with the disorder or "true positives") and specificity (the ability not to select those without the disorder or "true negatives") are considered to have the best accuracy in discriminating between patients and controls and, therefore, are favored as diagnostic criteria. In the ideal case, a specific organic marker, a *sign*, confirms a specific diagnosis and is referred to as a diagnostic "gold standard."

Of course, not all diseases or conditions have diagnostic gold standards. One can think of a continuum of diagnostic certainty ranging from diagnoses based on clear and present biophysical signs (either directly or indirectly visible through technoscientific methods) to those that rely heavily on descriptive and interpretive evidence. Although much everyday medical practice involves fairly unambiguous diagnostic work, of greatest sociological interest are those that fall on the latter end of this continuum. Because these descriptive diagnoses are often medically and socially contested, they raise interesting questions about biomedicine's contemporary cultural authority and power (Brown 1995).[6] In short, in the absence of clear biophysical evidence for disease, how and why are diagnoses constituted? The case of FMS is illustrative.

The Emerging Idea of Fibromyalgia Syndrome

The medical literature frequently suggests that fibromyalgia has existed throughout time. Biblical passages, as well as ancient medical references, are used to reveal the historical continuity of the disorder (Smythe 1989; Wallace and Wallace 1999). Despite this presumed ancient lineage, it is widely recognized that a few key publications concerning the rheumatic condition "fibrositis" in the 1970s marked a critical turning point in the contemporary framing of FMS.

Stage One: The (Re)introduction of Fibrositis

Fibrositis is a condition with a long history of medical marginality.[7] Sir William Gowers first introduced the term in 1904 in an article on lumbago in the *British Medical Journal.* The term "fibrositis," which means inflammation of fibrous tissue, was quickly judged erroneous; fibrous tissue cannot become inflamed. Nevertheless, the term persisted in medical parlance and was used to describe unexplainable, and ofttimes exaggerated, muscle and joint pain, including, for example, its application to shell-shocked soldiers in WWII. An article published in 1947 in the *Annals of Rheumatic Disease* argued that fibrositis be considered a form of "psychogenic rheumatism," given that those who suffered displayed no inflammation but had high rates of depression and anxiety (Boland 1947). This sentiment was widely adopted. During most of the twentieth century, fibrositis was essentially synonymous with psychogenic rheumatism, a belief that persisted and became entrenched in the minds of most physicians.

Such was the state of affairs in 1972 when rheumatologist Hugh Smythe wrote a chapter on fibrositis for the widely used textbook, *Arthritis and Allied Conditions.*[8] Smythe (1972) described fibrositis as a long-recognized and poorly understood rheumatic condition, but insisted that a distinct form of the disorder could easily be distinguished from that with psychogenic origins. In particular, unlike the *bizarre* forms of pain and paralysis seen with psychogenic rheumatism, Smythe contended that patients with fibrositis had truly *mundane* pain and that they could be distinguished by the presence of tenderness in characteristic locations. Smythe called these locations "tender points" and proposed that they be used as the key element in a set of diagnostic criteria to identify patients with fibrositis.[9]

The idea that tender places on the body are associated with muscular rheumatism has been propagated in various forms since the early 1900s. These tender places were called "nodules," "nerve points," "trigger points," and "tender points" by different researchers at different times during the twentieth century. As the existence of many different terms implies, a clear sense about the nature of these tender places and their biophysical existence has never been substantiated (Reynolds 1983). Nevertheless, Smythe employed the medically speculative concept of tender points to carve out a clinically identifiable pain syndrome from a collection of vague and diffuse symptoms described in the medical literature for at least two centuries.

By conceptually extracting a new and distinct medical entity from the residual category "psychogenic rheumatism," Smythe played a central entrepreneurial role in the diagnostic making of FMS. The response to Smythe's entrepreneurial effort was the burgeoning of fibrositis research as other clinician researchers eagerly set out to understand and treat this newly identified medical entity. Although Smythe's detailed description of fibrositis and his proposed criteria were significant, he had yet to test the criteria clinically. Was it possible to identify patients with fibrositis as Smythe suggested? Was there a subset of patients who could be conceptually disentangled from the amorphous category of psychogenic rheumatism? Answering these questions was the next stage in the diagnostic making of FMS.

Stage Two: The Entrepreneurial Challenge

During the 1980s, a small number of diagnostic entrepreneurs picked up where Smythe left off. The key players were four university-based rheumatologists: Muhammad Yunus (Peoria School of Medicine), Robert Bennett (Oregon Health Sciences University), Frederick Wolfe (University of Kansas School of Medicine), and Don Goldenberg (Boston University School of Medicine). Each had his own patients with ill-specified symptoms and multiple tender points as did Smythe's patients with fibrositis. This new cohort of diagnostic entrepreneurs favored the term "fibromyalgia". After all, their patients had no muscle and tissue inflammation and fibromyalgia better captured what they considered the disorder's cardinal symptom: muscle and joint pain. With a new name in hand, they set out to determine if it was possible to distinguish their patients with fibromyalgia from controls in clinical studies. Was fibromyalgia a clinical entity they could measure and study and, therefore, hope to treat?

Rheumatologists Yunus, Bennett, Wolfe, and Goldenberg, each with his respective research team, clinically tested and published fibromyalgia criteria. They used case-controlled clinical studies to find the precise combination of symptoms that best adjudicated between patients they identified as having fibromyalgia and controls. As the 1980s came to a close, however, the results of their collective research efforts were troubling and paradoxical. Each of the research teams published clinically tested FMS criteria, but their criteria differed. They all proposed tender points as criteria but disagreed about their location and how many were required for diagnosis. They also disagreed on which, if any, of the symptoms commonly associated with fibromyalgia (e.g., fatigue, sleep disorders, irritable bowel syndrome) were diagnostically necessary. The lack of consensus in establishing criteria fed into the well-entrenched sense that, whether the condition was called "fibrositis" or "fibromyalgia syndrome," it was an ill-specified diagnosis at best.

Stage Three: The American College of Rheumatology Criteria

To address the heterogeneity of existing criteria sets, the diagnostic entrepreneurs agreed to come together, collectively design and conduct a study, and identify the single best set of diagnostic criteria for fibromyalgia. Rheumatologists from a total of sixteen research centers joined their effort. This group, which became the American College of Rheumatology (ACR) Multicenter Fibromyalgia Criteria Committee, eventually proposed the fibromyalgia diagnostic criteria that were formally approved by the ACR.

In brief, the Committee research proceeded as follows. First, each of the participating research centers contributed a number of patients it identified as having fibromyalgia and a designated number of controls. To correct for earlier variations in data collection, researchers gathered standardized data on patients and controls at each participating center and then determined what factors best distinguished patients from controls. Based on a series of statistical combinations and comparisons, the Committee concluded that multiple tender points were the "most powerful discriminator between fibromyalgia patients and controls" (Wolfe et al. 1990: 166). In addition, they found that widespread pain (defined as pain in all four quadrants of the body) was found in 98 percent of patients with fibromyalgia, but in only 69 percent of controls. Whereas tender points had high levels of specificity, widespread pain was highly sensitive. The Committee combined these two features in its proposed criteria: eleven or more positive tender points (of eighteen test points), in combination with widespread pain, offered the most sensitive, specific, and accurate criteria for the diagnosis of FMS. Using these criteria, 88 percent of patients with fibromyalgia were identified as having fibromyalgia (true positives), and 81 percent of controls were identified as not having fibromyalgia (true negatives).

The ACR study, thus, established a category of patients who could be recognized in a clinical context with a high level of accuracy. Fibromyalgia, the Committee concluded, is an identifiable clinical entity, and the uniform diagnostic criteria it established were advanced and adopted by the ACR in 1990. The published account of the Committee's research appeared in *Arthritis and Rheumatism*, the official journal of the ACR.

Stage Four: FMS Post-ACR

Between 1972 and 1990 much and little had changed with respect to fibrositis syndrome. Smythe's initial specification of criteria in 1972 brought new attention to a common and poorly understood set of symptoms that had long brought a steady stream of patients to rheumatology and general outpatient clinics. His criteria were tested, modified, tested again, and eventually evolved into the fibromyalgia diagnostic criteria formally adopted by the ACR. But identifying criteria, formally adopting the diagnosis into medical nomenclature, and changing the disorder's name did not result in medical consensus. Despite the ACR Committee's best intentions to move beyond the contested history of psychogenic rheumatism and fibrositis, what remained the same, by any name, was the disorder's lack of an objective biomedical sign or marker.

The diagnosis of FMS is dependent on the subjective report of patients. Tender points do not represent fibrous tissue or muscle pathology and, therefore, do not represent anatomical pathology (Block 1999). The ACR Committee's elaborate analysis did not establish objective criteria. Instead it formalized a standard set of subjective criteria derived through clinical observation. Moreover, the ACR's analysis was built on a methodological flaw, set in motion by Smythe, and reproduced in every subsequent FMS diagnostic study. FMS is a *tautology*: tender points both define and substantiate its existence. Stated simply, the diagnostic entrepreneurs compared patients with FMS (defined by the presence of a large number of positive tender points) with controls (individuals without a large number of positive tender points) and found, over and again in study after study, that a large number of positive tender points best distinguished patients with FMS from controls.[10] According to one of the most outspoken FMS critics, although the ACR study generated no shortage of statistics, nothing could save it from having already "succumbed to a 'garbage in/garbage out' problem" (Bohr 1996: 594).

If FMS was not controversial enough, in 1992 a working group at the Second World Congress on Myofascial Pain and Fibromyalgia, which included many of the diagnostic entrepreneurs, proposed flexibility in the diagnostic criteria in a document titled the *Copenhagen Declaration*. An article in the British medical journal *Lancet* (Csillag 1992: 663–64) quotes from the *Copenhagen Declaration*:

> [T]he diagnosis is commonly entertained in the presence of unexplained widespread pain or aching, persistent fatigue, generalized [morning] stiffness, non-refreshing sleep, and multiple tender points. Most patients with these symptoms have 11 or more tender points. But a variable proportion of other typical patients may have less than 11 tender points at the time of the examination.

Thus, the group recommended clinical flexibility in the tender point requirement for patients who otherwise exhibit some of the symptoms that cluster as part of a wider syndrome: "encompassing headaches, irritable bladder, dysmenorrhoea, cold sensitivity, Raynaud's phenomenon, restless legs, atypical patters of numbness and tingling, exercise intolerance, and complaints of weakness" (Csillag 1992: 664).The recommendations outlined in the *Copenhagen Declaration* were subsequently incorporated into the World Health Organization's tenth edition of *International Statistical Classification of Disease and Related Health Problems* (1993). As a result, strictly speaking, there are no necessary or sufficient criteria (the tender point count can be flexible) or required number of associated symptoms (no particular number was specified in the *Copenhagen Declaration*) for FMS to exist. In practical terms, this opens the door for tremendous variation in how individual practitioners diagnose conditions in individual patients in clinical settings, leading some critics to argue that it is nearly impossible not to arrive at a diagnosis of FMS for *every* patient with widespread pain and tenderness of unknown origin (Cohen 1999).

These criticisms notwithstanding, FMS has been endowed with social life and that life continues to unfold. Favorably inclined rheumatologists and other medical practitioners have a new diagnosis for their dealings with a large and persistent patient population and millions of sufferers have now had their conditions diagnosed. The diagnostic making of FMS has also created a new professional niche of treatment and research. Diagnostic entrepreneur Robert Bennett summarizes the story thus far and, in so doing, outlines both the professional problems and promise FMS represents.

> Fibromyalgia is a clinical construct that has been developed, for the most part, by rheumatologists. It is a direct descendent of "fibrositis," a common misnomer that was first coined in 1904. There are always problems inherent in defining a disorder in purely descriptive terms. Nevertheless the publication of the American College of Rheumatology's 1990 Classification Criteria for fibromyalgia has been coincident with an impressive resurgence of research in this area (Bennett 2003: 5).

FMS: A Body of Knowledge[11]

Even before the ACR criteria were formally established, the efforts of the diagnostic entrepreneurs drew enough attention to promote interest among other clinician researchers. Slowly at first, but then with increasing pace, additional research appeared in the medical literature. By the end of 2000 more than 1,000 fibromyalgia publications appeared in the medical literature, most of them in one of thirteen rheumatology journals.[12] Figure 1.1 illustrates the historical trajectory of these publications, breaking them down by type: research articles (n = 627), review articles (n = 179), and comments or editorial pieces (n = 220).

As already outlined, the few publications in the early years focused primarily on describing the clinical entity of fibrositis and reflecting on its long history under various, now medically anachronistic, names such as psychogenic rheumatism and lumbago. The number of research publications picked up appreciably, beginning in the mid 1980s, as earlier descriptive work gave way to the second wave of diagnostic entrepreneurship, including the clinical testing of proposed diagnostic parameters. By the mid 1980s, these efforts prompted others to investigate the disorder's pathophysiology, etiology, and treatment. Correspondingly, from the mid 1980s onward, a substantial number of review articles appeared, indicating the emergence of an area or body of research considered worthy of systematic appraisal and critique. These trends become even more pronounced in the wake of the adoption of the ACR criteria in 1990. Finally, the steady rise in comment and editorial publications reveals the debate—assertions and counter-assertions concerning the scientific basis of the diagnosis and disorder—that has become increasingly intense.

One can summarize the divide within the body of FMS knowledge into two overarching positions. First, those who argue that FMS is an organic disorder or a disorder with a central organic component, and second,

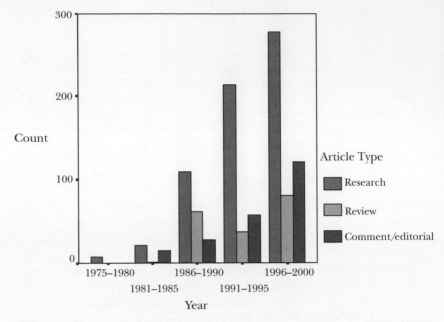

Figure 1.1   Fibromyalgia Publications in the Medical Literature, 1975–2000.

those who claim the disorder is a psychogenic or behavioral disorder, some of whom reject the scientific merit of the diagnosis itself. In practice, these camps are far from internally monolithic because extreme and moderate positions are found within each. Moreover, these camps are not truly mutually exclusive or exhaustive. Some researchers interpret FMS as a neurobiological psychiatric disorder, but suggest that current psychiatric classifications be used in lieu of the FMS diagnosis. Also blurring the division, very few in the organic camp would argue that psychological and behavioral factors play no role in FMS, and some attempt to bridge the organic/psychogenic divide by promoting a "biopsychosocial" account of FMS. Despite the complexity of positions, the crux of the debate over FMS is essentially a division between those who believe FMS is linked to some aberrant physiology and those who do not.

This divide can be seen in the FMS research literature. By far the most common types of FMS publications (almost half of all research articles) are those that explore factors thought to be associated, possibly causally, with FMS (see Appendix A for more details). Figure 1.2 illustrates the five most common factors studied in FMS association or causation research in terms of numbers of publications over time. Four of these are organic pursuits, whereas the fifth encompasses research testing a host of psychological

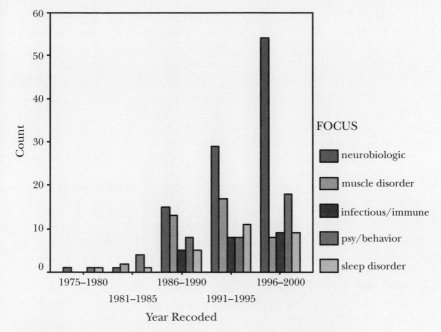

Figure 1.2 Focus of Fibromyalgia Publications, 1975–2000.

or behavioral hypotheses. The general knowledge claims of these camps will now briefly be summarized.

Organic Pursuits

Given the musculoskeletal nature of FMS pain, it is not surprising that significant effort has been directed toward finding abnormalities in muscle tissue of those who sufferer such pain. Studies in the 1980s looked promising. Some found evidence for structural irregularities in muscle and related soft tissue in patients with FMS, whereas others found the muscles of those with FMS to have diminished energy metabolism. These studies were poorly designed, however, and all subsequent attempts to find muscle abnormalities failed (Block 1999). The collective results from more than two decades of research demonstrate no muscle or soft tissue pathology, either in structure or performance, with FMS, although this has hardly curbed the efforts of some clinician researchers to prove otherwise (Block 1999).

Similarly persistent have been attempts to establish a link between sleep irregularities and FMS. In 1977, concurrent with his attempts to specify fibrositis criteria, Smythe and a colleague at the University of

Toronto published an account of fibrositis as "a non-restorative sleep syndrome" characterized by electroencephalograph (EEG) images of disturbed stage-4 or non–rapid eye movement (REM) sleep (Smythe and Moldofsky 1977). Since the 1970s, several studies have demonstrated differences in the brain wave activity in non-REM sleep of patients with FMS compared with healthy controls. One recent study found these abnormalities predictive of FMS-symptom severity (Roizenblatt et al. 2001). Although promising, these findings lack sensitivity and specificity; many individuals whose condition is diagnosed as FMS have no such abnormalities, and such abnormalities are both associated with other disorders and widely present in the general (healthy) public. After twenty-five years of ongoing research in this vein, no convincing evidence yet links FMS to any specific and objectively measurable sleep abnormalities (Cohen 1999). As with muscle pathology research, however, the lack of promising findings has not deterred researchers who continue to pursue links between FMS and sleep irregularities—perhaps spurred on by the fact that nearly all those whose condition is diagnosed as FMS report nonrestful sleep and morning fatigue (Abeles 1998).

Research exploring the link between FMS and infectious illness has also met with little success. More than two dozen review and research articles evaluating a possible association between infectious illness and FMS have been published, but no convincing link has been established (Goldenberg 1999). It is generally accepted that FMS does not have an immune component, although many sufferers associate the onset of their symptoms with a prolonged infectious illness and report an ongoing subjective sense of immune deficiency.[13] Once again, persistent, nonsupportive findings have not brought an end to this line of inquiry.

Figure 1.2 dramatically reveals the current emphasis of FMS research. An increasing number of clinician researchers argue that fibromyalgia is a neurobiological disorder. In contrast to the above-noted dead ends, this is currently the most promising organic account of the disorder. Several of the diagnostic entrepreneurs, including Bennett and Goldenberg, describe FMS as a disorder characterized by aberrant central pain processing. In particular, it is argued that individuals with FMS experience nonpainful stimuli as painful (called allodynia) and have an exaggerated response to painful stimuli (called hyperalgesia). It is assumed, therefore, that FMS involves an abnormality in nociception, the process by which painful stimuli are transmitted neurochemically between the peripheral and central nervous systems.

Several possible explanations have been advanced for why the body's system of pain perception malfunctions but, in general, they all involve various notions of neurochemical cross circuiting. Somewhere within the body's system for pain perception, which includes the peripheral nerves,

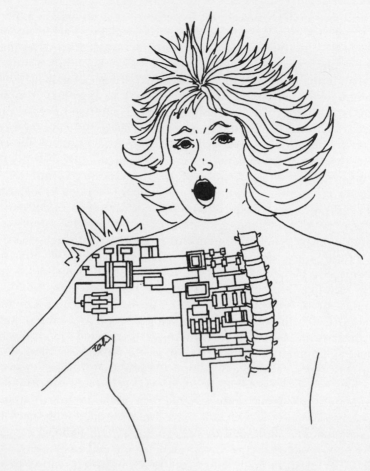

Figure 1.3 Graphic Depiction of Short-Circuiting (Wallace and Wallace 1999: xiv).

the spinal cord, the brain, and specific neurotransmitters, neurochemical misinformation is sent or processed. The body becomes hyperresponsive to pain, even in the absence of painful stimuli. Figure 1.3 from an FMS self-help book sponsored by the Arthritis Foundation, provides a simple visual representation of nociceptive malfunctioning (or a short-circuiting) in the central nervous system that results in an alteration in pain processing.

A leading explanation for why patients with FMS have such short-circuiting involves a phenomenon called "wind-up" (Bennett 1999b). In simple terms, wind-up is the neurochemical outcome of chronic pain. When pain lasts long enough and is intense enough, the argument goes, it tricks the body's neurochemistry into perceiving pain when there are no painful stimuli. Ordinarily, the experience of acute pain is in proportion to painful stimuli; when we get injured, we experience pain; as the injury heals, the pain too subsides. Researchers argue that this framework does not apply to *chronic* pain states wherein no direct link is found between an injury (painful stimuli) and the experience of pain. Therefore, rheumatologists are unable to trace pain back to any physical injury or anatomic pathology. Advocates of this stance claim that once the neuroscience of chronic pain states are more widely acknowledged by medical orthodoxy, fibromyalgia, which is said to occupy the far end of a spectrum of chronic pain, will no longer be controversial.

This model of FMS as a disorder of pain amplification is intuitively and culturally compelling. In addition, it accounts for the defining criterial feature of FMS: the characteristic presence of multiple tender points. A large number of tender points that respond to low levels of stimuli suggest an alteration in pain perception. But more persuasive yet, this model theoretically integrates empirical evidence purportedly demonstrating an association between FMS and neurobiological abnormalities.

For example, it is claimed that FMS is related to irregularities in two neurotransmitters involved in nocicpetion—serotonin and substance P. Metaphorically, neurotransmitters are understood as the brain's chemical messengers. As a neurotransmitter involved in the body's pain response, substance P sends pain signals to the spinal cord that, in turn, communicates the message of pain to the brain. Accordingly, too much substance P in the body could result in the perception of nonpainful stimuli as painful (allodynia) and an exaggerated response to painful stimuli (hyperalgesia). Several studies that have found elevated substance P levels in the spinal fluid of those with FMS are routinely marshaled in support of the neurobiological model. Although interesting, an elevation of substance P is found in many other conditions in which pain is a central feature and, therefore, is not specific to FMS (Cohen 1999).

Whereas substance P encourages the communication of pain messages to the brain, it is argued that the neurotransmitter serotonin helps regulate or discourage the message of pain. Therefore, too little serotonin (or diminished serotonin effect) could lead to fairly harmless stimuli being experienced as painful (hyperalgesia). In line with this argument, studies that have found an association between FMS and compromised serotonin levels and metabolism are heralded as additional proof of neurobiological causation (Russell et al. 1992). As will be explained shortly, however, others interpret these same findings as evidence that FMS is merely the somatic presentation of depression. Making the matter more complex yet, recent research has failed to replicate the association between serotonin uptake and fibromyalgia (Legangneux et al. 2001).

Other empirical evidence said to confirm the neurobiological basis of aberrant pain processing in FMS comes from reports of brain abnormalities detected through imaging technology. Researchers claim that FMS is characterized by single-photon emission computerized tomography (SPECT) images that show decreased blood flow to a location in the brain involved in nociception (Mountz et al. 1995). This research is criticized as being riddled with methodological flaws, most centrally involving the selection of appropriate controls (Abeles 1998). Research has yet to compare patients with FMS with other chronic pain patients. It is unclear, therefore, if the observed SPECT alterations are unique to FMS or common to pain states more generally. Moreover, these studies have not adequately controlled for psychiatric illness, even though SPECT alterations are all the rage in neuropsychiatry. Consequently, as with linking FMS to serotonin abnormalities, evidence of SPECT alterations can equally support the claim that FMS is principally a psychiatric condition.

In yet another vein, researchers assert that FMS involves neuroendocrine irregularities, in particular, dysregulation in the hypothalamus-pituitary-adrenal (HPA) axis (Crofford et al. 1996). In lay terms, the HPA axis is involved in the body's stress response. Individuals with FMS, it is argued, do not have a normal response to acute physical or psychological stress but, rather, their bodies behave as though they are in a chronic state of stress. This argument is based on observed alterations of certain neurohormones (growth hormone and cortisol) among those with FMS (Crofford and Clauw 2002; Goldenberg 1999). At question, however, are how these neuroendocrine abnormalities associated with stress are linked to FMS symptoms and what causes HPA dysregulation in the first place. For example, psychiatric distress can impact HPA functioning, leading other researchers to use these same findings in support of the psychogenic account of FMS (Abeles 1998).

Based on the combined neurobiological evidence (i.e., neurotransmitter and neurohormonal anomalies), some clinician researchers suggest that FMS is characterized by an abnormality in sensory processing more generally, called "central sensitivity," of which pain processing is but one aspect. A heightened response to a host of stimuli would account for many of the somatic complaints that make up the FMS symptom constellation. Likewise, it would account for the widely recognized overlap between FMS and other controversial syndromes involving sensory sensitivity, such as chronic fatigue syndrome (CFS), multiple chemical sensitive (MCS), irritable bowel syndrome (IBS), and premenstrual syndrome (PMS), to name but a few. Following this logic, some clinician researchers claim that, along with these other syndromes, fibromyalgia is best described as a *dysregulation spectrum syndrome* or a syndrome in which some common underlying mechanism manifests itself in hypersensitivity to a wide range of sensory stimuli (Yunus 2001: 130).

Even as many of the leading FMS clinician researchers promote an account of FMS as a dysregulation spectrum syndrome or a disorder of central sensory processing, few of them fail to acknowledge the *complex* nature of fibromyalgia, by which they mean the influence of nonbiological factors. Instead, they accept that an important interplay exists between the psychological, social, and biophysical aspects of FMS. Some have misappropriated the term "biopsychosocial" (Henriksson 2002),[14] whereas others suggest that FMS and related syndromes are "stress-associated" to capture the interplay between the body's biochemical stress response and the everyday lives of individuals (Crofford et al. 1996).

Although it would be false to say that the neurobiological perspective is monocausal, it is fair to say it frames FMS as *primarily* organic with associated psychological factors. For example, although Bennett himself maintains that one would be misguided to approach FMS as either a solely organic or solely psychological problem, it is clear that his orientation favors the former, as does his research agenda. The essence of this perspective, with its ambition to tie together sensory dysfunction and neurobiological abnormalities, is nicely captured in the following quote from Bennett's report, aptly titled *The Scientific Basis for Understanding Pain in Fibromyalgia:*

> Considering the preponderance of studies pointing to a dysfunction of sensory processing in fibromyalgia, one would expect these patients to have an amplification of bodily sensations resulting in a wide range of somatic symptoms. A diagnosis of somataform disorder [a disorder characterized by multiple symptoms that cannot be traced to a physical cause] will become a non-psychiatric diagnosis once the symptomology is adequately explained by disordered physiology (Bennett 2003: 1).

Psychopathological and Behavioral Pursuits

As a diagnostic subset carved out of the residual category of psychogenic rheumatism by Smythe and other diagnostic entrepreneurs, FMS was born under the burden of doubt. Consequently, when rheumatologists were unable to produce solid evidence of an organic basis for the new disorder, it took no time for a psychogenic framing of the disorder to crystallize and build over time (see Figure 1.2). Early on, some clinician researchers claimed that FMS symptoms were the somatic manifestation of psychological distress and they supported these claims with their anecdotal impressions that many of those whose conditions were diagnosed as FMS were mentally unwell. By the 1980s, clinician researchers began to test empirically the anecdotal sense that there was a link between FMS and psychological distress. A study in 1982 using the Minnesota Multiphasic Personality Inventory (MMPI) found that patients with FMS were more psychologically disturbed than patients with other painful rheumatic diseases (Payne et al. 1982). The fact that almost all of the thirty patients in the study had higher MMPI scales than controls led researchers to conclude that FMS is likely a psychological disturbance that has musculoskeletal pain as a principal symptom. This research was quickly attacked as methodologically flawed on two grounds. First, it was argued that the MMPI is not a meaningful measurement of psychological well-being for individuals experiencing chronic pain. Because pain is scored by the MMPI as an indicator of underlying depression, general pain symptoms could be wrongly captured by the MMPI as psychological distress. (This critique is weakened by the fact the controls were also pain patients, and so the inventory's distortion would have also found its way into their MMPI scores.) The study was also criticized for using hospitalized patients, who are likely to be more seriously ill than the average FMS sufferer. A more representative sample, for instance, would be patients with FMS seen on an outpatient basis.

Subsequent research using different methods, different indices of psychological well-being, and different patient and control populations made claims and counter-claims concerning the association between psychological distress and FMS: there is an association, there is not an association, and back and forth again. Despite the heated back-and-forth rhetoric, by the late 1980s, with several dozen studies in hand, it became clear to most commentators that there *is* an association between FMS and certain affective disorders, especially anxiety and major depressive disorder (Hudson and Pope 1989; Wolfe et al. 1984).

The link between FMS and depression is multifaceted. First, the symptoms of FMS and depression overlap: pain, fatigue, memory problems, and sleep irregularities. There are also high rates of comorbidity between the disorders: 50 to 70 percent of those with FMS have a history of depression. Third, low levels of antidepressant medications are among the most effective (of otherwise ineffective) medical treatments for FMS. Finally, as discussed above, the neurological findings that have been advanced as characteristic abnormalities of FMS, including serotonin metabolism and HPA axis dysregulation, are also characteristic of depression and anxiety (Hudson and Pope 1996).

Although the association between FMS and depression is now indisputable, as with everything else surrounding the FMS debate, simple facts have multiple interpretations. On one side are those who argue that the experience of FMS *results* in psychopathology as a secondary or side effect. This position is intuitively appealing, given that enduring years of debilitating and unexplainable symptoms would likely cause psychological distress in many, if not most, individuals. Most of the diagnostic entrepreneurs claim that when anxiety and depression are present they are generally the result, not the cause, of FMS (Goldenberg 1999; Yunus 1991). Undercutting this analysis are studies that demonstrate that psychopathology pre-dates the onset of FMS in most cases (Hudson and Pope 1996). Alternatively, FMS could be the *effect* of psychiatric distress; the symptoms could be a somatic presentation of depression. This position also has logical merit, given the shared symptoms and neurochemical abnormalities of both disorders, but not all individuals with FMS have demonstrable psychopathology, which critically weakens this position. A third stance, somewhere in between these poles, proposes that FMS and depression are linked via another, shared but unknown, pathology (Hudson and Pope 1989; Hudson and Pope 1996).

In sum, the straightforward association between FMS and depression turns out to be anything but straightforward. Does FMS cause depression? Does depression manifest itself as FMS symptoms? Or, are FMS symptoms and depression linked by some third condition? Current research is simply unable to answer this question with any degree of certainty. In the absence of a definitive answer, the high rates of depression among those who suffer from FMS (who otherwise have no consistent biological abnormality) result in persistent claims that FMS is best understood as a mental, not a physical illness.

Research showing an overlap between FMS and the psychiatric diagnosis post-traumatic stress disorder (PTSD) is also used to bolster this claim. The PTSD diagnosis was introduced in the Diagnostic and Statistical Manual of Mental Disorders, Third Edition (DSM-III) published in 1980 and, at that time, was still associated primarily with combat experience (in particular, service in Vietnam). Over time, however, the diagnosis has applied to a more diverse population of trauma "survivors," most especially victims of sexual and physical abuse. In one study, nearly 60 percent of patients with FMS had "clinically significant levels of PTSD symptoms," a prevalence rate significantly higher than in the general population (Cohen et al. 2002: 38). From the other direction, a study of patients with PTSD found high rates of undiagnosed FMS: 21 percent of those with PTSD also met the criteria for FMS, whereas none of the individuals in a relevant control group met the criteria for FMS (Amir et al. 1997).

These studies, along with several others, reveal a significant overlap between FMS and PTSD, using the existing diagnostic standards of each disorder. Nevertheless, the existence of this association does not amount to a clear victory for the psychogenic camp. As with FMS, the scientific merits of the PTSD diagnosis have been called into question (Young 1995). Thus, there is uncertainty about exactly what it means to observe an overlap in two problematic diagnoses. Independent of the PTSD diagnosis, a few studies address the possible link between FMS and sexual, physical, and emotional abuse. Some found an association between FMS and childhood or adult abuse, as well as an association between the severity of FMS symptoms and abuse history, but no clear causal link has been established (Boisset-Pioro et al. 1995; Taylor et al. 1995; Walker et al. 1997). As a whole, current research charting the relationship between FMS, PTSD, and childhood or adult abuse raises more questions than it answers.

Some of the most vocal opponents of the diagnosis argue that FMS is not a defensible scientific concept at all; rather, it represents a type of illness behavior in which psychologically unstable individuals, having exhausted their ability to cope, become hyperaware of their symptoms and tirelessly seek out physicians willing to give a medical label to a cluster of psychological problems (Bohr 1996; Ehrlich 2003; Hadler 1999). Further, it is argued that patient support groups spread misinformation through the media (especially the Internet), thus spreading FMS along the way. Critics point out that all of this takes place in the context of disability and health care insurance systems that require patients to prove they are sick. Consequently, once this path has been initiated, sickness begets sickness or, in the words of Norton Hadler (1996: 2397), "If you have to prove you are ill, you can't get well." Insofar as FMS is an iatrogenic illness (an illness inadvertently induced by physicians), critics claim that labeling patients increases their level of sickness and associated social and economic costs.

These sweeping assertions are not readily supported empirically. The few studies attempting systematically to assess their merit have not been particularly convincing. As already noted, many of those whose condition is diagnosed as FMS do not exhibit psychopathology nor do they have exaggerated levels of psychological distress (Wolfe 1999). Likewise, claims that the FMS diagnosis is more disabling than enabling are mainly anecdotal conjecture and difficult to substantiate. FMS supporters maintain that patients find the label profoundly reassuring, which, in turn, results in a decrease in costly specialty referrals and diagnostic work-ups (Clements et al. 1997; Goldenberg 1999). The most sophisticated study on the topic to date, found that patients with newly diagnosed FMS report a significant improvement in their well-being and no significant differences in their rates of health care utilization or disability claims over a three-year period or in comparison with the period prior to diagnosis. In sum, the label did not appear to have a long-term negative effect on clinical outcome (White et al. 2002: 260).

A recent study assessing the prevalence of FMS among the Amish also challenges the claim that FMS is a type of illness behavior encouraged through ill-informed media coverage and a liberal system of disability compensation and insurance (White and Thompson 2003). The Amish do not have access to electronic media nor do they read any materials produced by non-Amish sources. In addition, the Amish do not use any public or private compensation systems and their strong work ethic discourages seeking financial assistance even through an established local process. All the same, 7.3 percent of an Amish community met the ACR tender point criteria, a rate significantly higher than among either urban or rural controls (3.8 and 1.2 percent, respectively). This study was quickly attacked as politically motivated in a series of editorials. One critic proposed that the dramatic results were likely attributable to biased tender point examinations given by over-zealous advocates of the FMS diagnosis—the more you believe, the harder you press, the more fibromyalgia you find—just proving that FMS "has become a social and political issue" (Wolfe 2003: 1671). Another critic noted that the diagnosis is effectively meaningless in the Amish context, because these individuals will not join support groups that perpetuate a sense of common misery, seek to have their disability affirmed, and generally "turn a common symptom into a remunerative industry" (Ehrlich 2003: 1666). In the minds of critics, this study merely found that the Amish have a high number of tender points, which is not to say they are a part of what we understand, either socially or medically, to be the FMS phenomenon.

From a less polemic stance, some of the complexities showcased in the above exchange are also addressed by clinician researchers who approach FMS from a biopsychosocial perspective. The term "biopsychosocial" is used by different researchers to mean very different things (see endnote 14), but its unique contribution is drawing attention to the important behavioral component of FMS. In particular, this perspective recognizes certain biological alterations (e.g., neurotransmitter and neurohormonal anomalies) in some patients with FMS, but rejects the idea that FMS is principally a biological abnormality and, instead, emphasizes the perception and response of individuals to common stresses (Masi et al. 2002). In essence, this approach takes as a given the ubiquity of pain, fatigue, and so forth, and frames FMS as a set of maladaptive physical, emotional, and behavioral responses to common symptoms.

Not unlike the organic neurobiological account, the psychopathological and behavioral accounts of FMS assume that patients misperceive or respond abnormally to physical or psychological stress. But, whereas the former suggests that sensory stimuli are misperceived as a result of neurochemical hypersensitivity, the latter account suggests a patient's hypervigilance results in misperceiving normal physical and psychological stresses, which then, in turn, confirms the patient's subjective sense of sickness. Distressed patients effectively see more symptoms and perceive them to be more serious. This, it is argued, accounts for the vast number of symptoms patients with FMS report, as well as the overlap between FMS and other contested illness (e.g., CFS, MCS) characterized by a host of somatic complaints. Along with FMS, it is asserted that these contested syndromes likely represent a shared or similar psychiatric condition characterized by hypervigilance and a corresponding tendency to somatize. For this reason, these functional somatic disorders are considered *affective spectrum disorders* by many clinician researchers.

The FMS Stalemate and Rheumatology's Dilemma

Parallels between the organic and psychogenic-behavioral accounts of FMS are pronounced and yet their divergent interpretations of similar facts and realities are striking. Despite the certainty with which each camp makes its claims, there is no way to adjudicate between their conflicting interpretations of the same evidence. It is currently impossible for the tools of biomedicine to distinguish between hyperalgesia and hypervigilance, making the arguments between the *dysregulation spectrum syndrome* and the *affective spectrum disorder* camps not resolvable. Whether the disorder has an organic basis, is a set of symptoms subsumable under existing psychiatric categories, is an iatrogenic phenomenon, or is some union between physical symptoms and maladaptive behavior has simply not been answered and may not be answerable even by well-designed studies. Accordingly, Micha Abeles (1998: 44) describes the various pathogenic hypotheses for FMS as a "babel of claims and counter claims." Her damning assessment is worthy of quoting at length.

> [C]ontending and competing hypotheses regarding causation is prima facie evidence of how little is actually known about FMS. Persistent promulgation of pet theories does not necessarily reflect credibility. Phenomenon and epiphenomenon are often confused or ignored, conflicting findings discarded and competing thoughts disregarded. Muscle pathology continues to be evoked, although clearly not present. Serotonin deficiency and substance P elevation have not been thoroughly enough studied to indicate what role (if any) they play in the symptoms of FMS. Disordered sleep patterns and accompanying alpha EEG anomalies occur in FMS but are not universal and are also seen in a variety of other vague disorders of fatigue and even in normal individuals. Depression is not an uncommon finding in FMS patients but does not explain the etiology of FMS in those with normal psychological profiles. Stress intensifies symptoms in FMS but its etiological role and the role of any neurohormonal changes associated with stress in the relationship to FMS is purely conjectural. . . . Why generalized pain is the end result of multiple unrelated processes remains an enigma.

The FMS debate, thus, begins and ends with the enigmatic character of pain and rheumatology's attempts to give it biomedical representation. But now, rheumatology finds itself awkwardly positioned vis-à-vis the efforts of the diagnostic entrepreneurs and the controversies those efforts have engendered. Patients with unexplainable pain and other distressing symptoms will fill rheumatology clinics as they have since Ralph Pemberton opened the first U.S. clinic for rheumatic conditions in 1926. There is no debating the fact that widespread pain and other distressing, common, and nonspecific symptoms currently gathered together under the diagnostic label FMS are a reality every rheumatologist faces. Many of the patients presenting these symptoms meet the FMS criteria. Because the elusive character of pain is exceeded only by patients' desire for its explanation and physicians' aspirations, when possible, to provide one, some practitioners see the FMS diagnosis as an invaluable addition to rheumatology's clinical toolbox for the management of this difficult-to-treat patient population.

The practical appeal likely explains why, on average, rheumatologists are more likely to be sympathetic to the FMS diagnosis than other medical practitioners (White et al. 2000). Nevertheless, many rheumatolgists express frustration both at the FMS diagnosis and with patients with FMS (Crofford and Clauw 2002; Gordon 2003). A 2002 editorial gives a long list of possible reasons for this discontent.

> The most simplistic reason for this frustration may be psychological distress on the part of patients, physicians, or both. Patients with FM display higher average levels of distress than do individuals with other rheumatic disorders. Previous unsatisfactory interactions with the health care system may increase the likelihood of an adversarial relationship between patient and physician. Distress on the part of physicians is likely because mechanisms underling FM symptoms are poorly understood and are outside of the realm of mechanisms traditionally studied by rheumatologists (e.g., immunology, inflammation, connective tissue biology). In addition, current pharmacologic therapies are often ineffective, nonpharmacologic therapies require time to implement, and dealing with contentious issues surrounding FM such as disability compensation or litigation is frustrating and counterproductive (Crofford and Clauw 2002: 1137).

Even one of the diagnostic entrepreneurs has become highly critical of what has become of FMS. According to Frederick Wolfe (2003), more than just "frustrating and counterproductive," one of the principal problems is relying on a purely descriptive category for determining legal matters such as public and private disability eligibility and worker's compensation. This same concern was rather sardonically expressed in a recent letter in the *Journal of Rheumatology* (Silva 2004: 828) that offered a scripted response for rheumatologists to follow when providing legal testimony concerning FMS disability and compensation:

Does the patient have fibromyalgia?

No one can have fibromyalgia. Fibromyalgia is just a word we use to represent the situation of someone complaining about widespread chronic pain, fatigue, and sleep disturbance who has tender points on physical examination. It is not a disease, it's a description.

This script also foreshadows another concern expressed by Wolfe and others, namely, the peculiarity of some researchers' seemingly undaunted commitment to nailing down the biophysicality of FMS. Such efforts, he notes, fail to acknowledge the possibility that the "Emperor is unclothed" (Wolfe 1999). As is made evident in their research agendas, some rheumatologists treat FMS as a material "thing" rather than an abstraction of their own making.

Wolfe blames the ACR criteria for both the legal dilemmas confronting rheumatology and the epistemological absurdity characteristic of current FMS research. In effect, he argues, the tender point examination is "disease-creating," because it gives undue weight to what is purely an intellectual construct and, thus, makes FMS seem mainly like a "physical disease" (Wolfe 2003: 1671). Consequently, Wolfe recommends that the ACR criteria should no longer be used, either in the clinic or for research purposes. Yet, Wolfe has not turned his back on the FMS diagnosis, conducting FMS research, or treating patients with FMS. Instead, he calls on rheumatologists to rely on more interpretative methods to diagnose FMS, including recording and listening to the breadth of patients' symptoms and suffering and, when possible, to "try to help" (Wolfe 2003: 1672).

Apart from the ambivalent views of rheumatology's rank and file or those of a maverick diagnostic entrepreneur, rheumatology's professional leadership has never been enthusiastic about FMS, and it appears as if any enthusiasm it may once have had is on the wane. Although dramatic when considered in isolation and in terms of its impact, the small number of FMS publications relative to the enormity of the FMS clinical population is testament to its marginality. Although fibromyalgia is one of the most common rheumatological disorders, the two most influential rheumatology journals—*Arthritis and Rheumatism* and *British Journal of Rheumatology*—have devoted only 1 percent of their manuscripts to the disorder since 1995 and both are publishing fewer such manuscripts now than five years ago (Goldenberg and Smith 2003). The professional leadership has also publicly suggested that rheumatology back away from its affiliation with FMS and its treatment. For example, in his 2001 ACR presidential address,

Michael Weinblatt (2002) recommended that, given the small number of rheumatologists and the large number of patients with well-established rheumatic conditions, the treatment of those with fibromyalgia is a less than ideal use of scarce resources. Implicit in the paucity of FMS publications and Weinblatt's remarks is the sense that little professional gain will come of rheumatology's intimate alliance with a contested diagnosis and an illness that shows little or no response to conventional medical interventions. In short, in the eyes of the leadership of an already struggling medical subfield, affiliation with a contested illness is seen as an ill-advised strategy of professional advancement.

Rheumatology's professional anxiety and guardianship over the organic-psychogenic divide is more than mere scientific chauvinism on the part of its leadership. Research funding options, as well as treatment compensation, are determined by where the objects of one's professional expertise fall on the organic-psychogenic continuum, as, in turn, does the ability of the field to draw the best and the brightest of the next generation of clinician researchers. The professional status of rheumatology, as with that of any medical specialty, is ultimately a function of its ability to claim expertise over organic illnesses.

For this reason, many of the diagnostic entrepreneurs and a new generation of FMS researchers push on in their efforts to establish the disorder's underlying organic mechanisms and, thereby, finally legitimate the controversial entity as well as their own professional agenda. Consequently, at the same time that rheumatology's professional leadership hopes to create some much needed distance between the subspecialty and FMS, a cadre of rheumatologists remains committed to preserving rheumatology's leading role in the biomedical understanding and treatment of FMS (Crofford and Clauw 2002; Goldenberg and Smith 2003). For good or ill, having created the diagnosis, provided a diagnosis to millions of sufferers, and launched a new area of biomedical research, rheumatology is inextricably linked to the controversial construct of fibromyalgia.

A Unique Story?

Before proceeding, it is important to put the FMS story into perspective. Although there are unique chapters in the FMS story, there are also ways in which it tells a more general tale about the relationship between contemporary society and biomedicine. Aspects of medical uncertainty surrounding FMS are not unique to it alone or even to contested diagnoses more generally. Many widely accepted disorders are also characterized by uncertainties. Many other conditions lack diagnostic precision or are difficult to diagnosis (e.g., asthma, osteoarthritis, rheumatoid arthritis) and, yet, the medical community accepts these conditions. Likewise, there are other disorders whose causal mechanisms are poorly understood or unknown (e.g., lupus, multiple sclerosis, scoliosis, allergies) and they, too, are acknowledged as legitimate medical conditions. In addition, the lack of efficacious treatment hardly sets FMS apart. Many conditions respond very poorly or only marginally to medical therapeutics (e.g., Alzheimer's disease, pancreatic cancer, acne) and, yet, these disorders are not discredit as "unreal" on such grounds.

Thus, many accepted disorders are plagued by some, or even significant, medical uncertainty. Of course, some of these conditions can hardly be in doubt, given that they dramatically and unambiguously manifest themselves in bodily disfigurement or the death of the sufferer. But others are neither disfiguring nor deadly. Whether fatal or not, there is a tremendous range in what medicine knows and does not know about any number of conditions. Moreover, not always does a consistent relationship exist between knowledge and effective treatment: there are conditions about which medicine knows a good deal but treats poorly, and others about which it knows very little but treats well. What is certain is that imperfect medical knowledge is ubiquitous to contemporary biomedicine.

Hence, one might argue that FMS and other contested diagnoses are but exaggerated or extreme cases of biomedicine's inevitable encounter with uncertainty. Whereas such uncertainty is hardly new, scholars have plausibly argued that more and more medical practice has become less and less precise, definitive, and firmly grounded (de Swaan 1989; Frank 1995; Ong 1995; Oudshoorn 1997). To a large degree, this can be attributed to the inherent difficulties many chronic conditions pose to the conventional biomedical theories and practices that proved far more effective in making sense of, and slaying, our earlier infectious enemies. But this alone is not the full story. Biomedicine's lack of certitude about contemporary illnesses is also the result of its engagement with an ever-expanding range of complex human distresses. On both counts, uncertainty grows as patients and clinicians alike seek to frame multifaceted forms of human suffering within the confines of the conventional biomedical model.

Although this story is focused on rheumatology and the making of FMS, it is also a story about what might be called our "postmodern" biomedical condition. By this I mean the situation in which we live with an increasing number of long-term afflictions that are ever more medically diffuse and elusive at the same time that their consequences for our quality of life are unmistakably tangible. Rheumatology's creation of FMS puts into sharp relief our cultural response to this larger dilemma.

2

The Woman Problem and the Feminization of Fibromyalgia Syndrome

The previous chapter summarized how rheumatologists developed the construct or idea of fibromyalgia syndrome (FMS) and the subsequent knowledge claims and counter-claims about that idea. Yet, the astute reader should be curious about a fact that is all but absent from this summary—absent because it is, in fact, conceptually absent from the knowledge and debate about FMS. The fact is that most of the millions of patients with FMS are women. Indeed, perhaps the single most interesting observation about the body of FMS knowledge is the virtual absence of any reference to sex, despite the disorder's overwhelming feminization.

Although studies conducted in different settings generate different estimates regarding the female-to-male ratio of those who meet the criteria for FMS, it is highly feminized. An estimate generated in a clinical rheumatology setting suggests the ratio is as high as 20:1, whereas one community-level study found the ratio to be as low as 3:1 (Bennett 1999; White et al. 1999). These differences in clinical and community ratios draw attention to the gender difference between patient and nonpatient populations, but they can also be taken as the extreme endpoints in a continuum of plausible sex-ratio estimates. A frequently cited statistic is that FMS is more prevalent among women than among men by a ratio of roughly 9:1, or approximately 90 percent of those who meet the FMS criteria are women (Hawley and Wolfe 2000). Notwithstanding the complexities associated with accurately determining the sex ratio of FMS, nearly every clinician knows that FMS is a disorder that primarily affects women.

As we have seen, however, the focus and trajectory of FMS research appears peculiarly disjointed from this fact. This chapter explores what I call the "present absence" of sex and gender from the idea of FMS. The central claim of this chapter is that FMS represents an attempt on the part of rheumatologists to put into biomedical language women's broadly felt somatic distress; yet, in the process of translating this distress into a biomedical abstraction, the gendered basis of the abstraction was, and indeed remains, obscured. Consequently, this chapter analytically highlights the gendered character of an illness not currently conceptualized through the lens of gender. Lastly, this chapter concludes that FMS is an example of a broader tendency—the distortion that emerges from the intersection of the complexity of women's somatic complaints and biomedical practice.

The Present Absence of Sex and Gender

The dearth of research exploring or seeking to explain the empirically undeniable association between women and FMS is remarkable. For example, of the 806 FMS research and review articles published through 2000, only eight explicitly address, as their primary focus, sex-related variables (e.g., sex hormones, menstruation, pregnancy, silicone breast implants) and their association with FMS.[1] Three additional articles describe the clinical differences in FMS symptomology between women and men; however, these studies do not centrally address the disorder's association to sex-related variables (Buskila et al. 2000; Wolfe et al. 1995a; Yunus et al. 2000). Also telling is that none of these eleven publications is a review article—a form of commentary that typically signals the recognition of an established body of medical research.[2] Judged on the basis of the existing medical literature, the relationship between FMS and what historian Thomas Laqueur (1990) calls the "sexed body" is most certainly *not* a central and explicit theme in the FMS biomedical research.

Moreover, applying the conceptual distinction between sex (biology) and gender (culture) to the FMS literature, it is evident also that FMS research does not direct attention to gender or gender differences to make sense of the feminization of FMS. Some research has found an association between FMS and various social–psychological characteristics (e.g., poor coping and stress management, low self-esteem, low self-efficacy), but this research did not draw on scholarship showing gender differences in these characteristics (or the gender bias in the conceptualization of these characteristics) (Rieker and Bird 2000; Rieker and Jankowski 1995). Additionally, a few studies have explored the relationship between FMS and sexual, physical, and emotional abuse, which, although not limited to women, are considered more common among them (see Chapter 1). Given biomedicine's overwhelmingly biological orientation, the trivial attention paid to cultural (gender) differences between men and women in FMS research is not all that surprising. We might, however, have expected a stronger focus on biological sex differences.

In contrast with the paucity of sex/gender research in the FMS literature, articles that explore the link between FMS and neurobiological abnormalities, muscle pathology, and psychopathology predominate.[3] As noted in the preceding chapter, the link between FMS and muscle pathology is considered a dead end by most clinician researchers, and the number of such research articles is rapidly on the decline. Articles that examine neurobiological and psychogenic-behavioral bases of FMS, on the other hand, are increasing in number. To date, these accounts of FMS remain highly provisional and leave much to be explained; however, one fact these accounts have made no attempt to explain is the overwhelming feminization of the disorder.

For example, researchers who embrace the interpretation of FMS as a pain amplification disorder resulting from an abnormality in the way painful stimuli are transmitted neurochemically occasionally note that women's lower pain threshold might account for their overrepresentation among those with FMS. They do not, however, follow this through in terms of specifying possible sex-linked processes or mechanisms underlying nociceptive alternation. Moreover, the current understanding of the role of sex in the neurochemistry of pain is still in its infancy and, therefore, unable to provide a definitive account for the feminization of FMS or other pain disorders in which women predominate (Berkley 1992; Fillingim 2000). Likewise, the stress-associated neurohormonal account of FMS simply does not implicate sexual dimorphism. The hypothalamus-pituitary-adrenal (HPA) axis is "upstream," so to speak, from circulating sex hormones and nothing about the currently hypothesized HPA axis dysregulation in FMS overlaps or intersects with sex differences. What is more, the greater claim that FMS represents a disorder in sensory processing more generally is not theoretically and conceptually linked to sex differences. In sum, current neurobiological claims about FMS, including that it represents a dysregulation spectrum syndrome, offer no explanation for the feminization of the disorder.

Psychogenic and behavioral accounts of FMS are similarly inattentive to the disorder's feminization. The overrepresentation of women among those with depression and anxiety is well documented and, by occasionally acknowledging this reality, the psychogenic account of FMS indirectly addresses the disorder's feminization.[4] No clear explanations exist, however, for women's overrepresentation among those with affective disorders in the general psychiatric literature; the role of reproductive hormones on the neurotransmitters that control mood remains speculative at best (Steiner et al. 2003). Among psychiatric researchers, a vigorous and unresolved debate exists concerning the intersecting role of sex and gender in women's affective illness states, including claims that psychiatric classifications themselves are sex biased (Rieker and Jankowski 1995; Umberson et al. 1996). Thus, to the extent that the psychogenic and affective spectrum disorder perspectives account for the feminization of FMS at all, they do so only by appealing to other disorders whose feminization remains unexplained. Finally, the various accounts of FMS that emphasize the role of maladaptive illness behavior in FMS are disconnected from any theoretical discussion about how and why such behaviors might account for the feminization of the disorder, despite a rich literature on gender differences in illness behavior (Hibbard and Pope 1986; Rieker and Bird 2000). Consequently, none of the existing accounts of FMS provides an explanation for the feminization of the disorder, nor has the feminization of the disorder been used as a rationale to shape the direction and development of FMS research. After more than two decades of committed research, the biomedical understanding of FMS is still tenuous and highly contentious. There are no objective indictors of the disorder nor are there clear theoretical accounts for what causes the disorder. There is disagreement about its pathogenic characteristics, and there are no genuinely effective treatment options. The almost total absence of sex or gender from the framing of FMS, therefore, is all the more peculiar, given that perhaps the only uncontested fact about this highly contested disorder is its feminization.

The absence of sex from FMS knowledge is also profoundly inconsistent with decades of feminist scholarship that compellingly argues that medical accounts of women's "natural" bodies have been infused by, and have served to reproduce, ideological assumptions about women's secondary status (Laqueur 1990; Newman 1985). A rich tradition of scholarship demonstrates how early scientific medical thought defined women's bodies as sexed *sine qua non* when seen through the presumed universality of the medical (male) norm. Historically, medicine has defined women's normal reproductive physicality as unstable and defined women's illnesses primarily in terms of their reproductive bodies (Ehrenreich and English 1973; Martin 1987; Martin 1991). Late 19th and early 20th century physicians, for example, not only assumed that the female reproductive body was the likely etiological culprit for women's maladies, but they also assumed that the female reproductive body was the very essence of *woman* (Newman 1985; Smith-Rosenberg 1985; Wood 1984). Medically speaking, women were the weaker sex; unlike men, their very being was dictated by their reproductive physicality. Although it is tempting to see such tendencies as relics from the past, feminist scholars have persuasively argued that contemporary biomedicine is still steeped in this tradition, as evidenced by its continued propensity to focus on women's reproductive bodies as the likely source of women's medical problems (Clarke and Olesen 1999; Martin 1987; Oudshoorn 1994).

Consequently, we might have expected FMS research to be replete with accounts of how yet another female malady can be traced to women's unruly and unstable, reproductive sexed bodies. We might have expected FMS research to offer a thinly veiled biological justification for women's secondary status—proof that women's social ambitions are often thwarted by physical limitations and incompatible with their innate character. Instead, biologically sexed bodies are almost entirely absent from the FMS research literature.

A straightforward explanation for a lack of biomedical interest in the link between sex and FMS would be that research in the area has proved fruitless and so directed clinician researchers to look elsewhere. It is difficult to sustain this argument, given the very small number of studies exploring the sex-FMS link in the first place. In addition, of these very few studies, most used methodologies that fail to offer any clarity on questions concerning the link between sex and FMS. For example, researchers in three separate studies asked women to assess, retrospectively, the onset and severity of their FMS symptoms in relationship to menstruation, pregnancy, or menopause (Ostensen et al. 1997; Raphael and Marbach 2000; Waxman and Zatzkis 1986). In each of these studies, researchers inferred that a likely association exists between sex hormones and FMS, because women subjectively "recall" a connection between their symptoms and events characterized by sex hormone fluctuation. Two less-speculative studies explored the relationship between sex hormones and FMS, but they came to different conclusions. One found that during the postovulatory phase of the menstrual cycle, women with FMS (compared with controls) exhibited a lower level of a particular neurochemical involved in pain perception, suggesting that sex hormones might play a role in FMS (Anderberg et al. 1998). A second study found that women with FMS and chronic fatigue syndrome (CFS) did not demonstrate abnormalities in gonadal steroid levels as part of a neuroendocrine stress response (Korszun et al. 2000: 1526). In combination, existing research on the role sex plays in FMS is sparse and inconclusive. At the same time, one would be hard pressed to argue that research pursuits unrelated to sex have been so encouraging as to make all other paths appear irrelevant.

That biomedicine has avoided framing FMS as intrinsically connected to the vagaries of women's bodies and their resultant constitutional frailty, in many regards, is progressive. It could possibly indicate an ideological shift within medicine itself—one that assumes a less-biased orientation regarding the link between women's reproductive bodies and their health. Nevertheless, the current framings of FMS are not yielding coherent and promising answers and treatments and, with so many unanswered questions, the failure to put the overwhelming feminization of the disorder to intellectual use is puzzling. Why has FMS not been conceptually framed as a women's health issue? Why and how is it that women are simultaneously present but absent from our current thinking about FMS? To explore these questions, we begin by turning to the relevant theoretical and substantive literature on women's health.

The Impact of Sex and Gender on Women's Health and Illness

Margaret Mead's *Sex and Temperament in Three Primitive Societies*, published in 1935, and Simone de Beauvoir's *The Second Sex*, published in 1952, laid the early groundwork for modern, sometimes called "second wave," feminist thought. In particular, they explicitly theorized the conceptual distinction between sex and gender and therefore made possible a political project premised on a rejection of the inherent or fixed *nature* of women's inequality. Whereas sex includes the biological distinctions between male and female, gender entails the social–cultural meanings and implications of being a man or woman. Sex differences include variations in chromosomes, gonads, hormones, and secondary sex characteristics. In contrast, gender differences include differential access to scarce resources and the corresponding social practices, identities, and ideologies that emerge from, and structure, those inequalities. Since the landmark treatises of Mead and de Beauvoir, feminists have had much to say about sex, gender, and their relationship to one another, but, for now, we will proceed by drawing on the above-noted distinction as it relates to women's health.

Making the distinction between sex and gender is helpful in that it allows us to distinguish, at least conceptually, between the effects of biology and culture on women's health. Historically and cross-culturally, there have been, and are, differences in the health and well-being of women and men. Even though we see variations in health by sex in all past and present societies, the character of these variations differ. Indeed, the variable effects of sex on health across time and space suggest that inherent sex differences alone are an insufficient explanation for observed health disparities between women and men. This implicates the effects of gender on health status: gender relations in a given time and place necessarily mediate the relationship between sex and health.

Although gender is culturally ubiquitous, it does not have a uniform or universal impact on the well-being of all women or all men, even in a given time and place. Rather, the impact of gender identities, practices, and structures on the health of women and men varies, depending on class, race, ethnicity, age, and sexual orientation. Nevertheless, gender influences women's health in ways that warrants theoretical consideration. Lesley Doyal (1995: 7), for example, notes that, despite differences among women, they "share the reality of occupying (more or less) subordinate positions in most social and cultural contexts" and this gendered reality has important consequences for women's health.

The Women's Health Paradox

In the United States and other industrializing nations, women lived shorter lives than men into the nineteenth century. Before that, frequent pregnancies, high maternal mortality, and short life expectancies characterized the lives of most women. But, by the mid 1800s, men's mortality advantage began to erode as women's fertility and maternal mortality rates declined. Consequently, by the end of the nineteenth century, a pronounced pattern in health statistics crystallized that persists to this day: women outlive men. In 1900, they did so by only three years; by 1950, they did so by approximately five years; today, they do so in excess of seven years. Even though black women have lower life expectancy than white women, their mortality advantage relative to black men is even more dramatic: they outlive their black male counterparts by more than eight years (National Center for Health Statistics 2000).[5]

Even as women in the United States have a mortality advantage over men, they have significantly higher, age-adjusted morbidity, or rates of illness. This is seemingly paradoxical. Women's mortality advantage would seem to imply a general health advantage over men. Nevertheless, their comparative robustness with respect to mortality does not translate into greater health vitality overall. Women experience a disproportionate burden of nonfatal acute and chronic aliments, pain, and dysfunction. They report more sick days than men, as well as more workdays lost to disability. They have more health care visits (even controlling for reproductive health care), higher prescription and over-the-counter drug use, and they report significantly more physical discomfort and limitation. In addition, women consistently evaluate their mental health less favorably than men: they have higher rates of self-reported emotional and psychological distress as well as more mental health consultations (Doyal 1995).[6] Using any number of different indicators of well-being, women live longer but are sicker and more disabled than men (Verbrugge 1990; Verbrugge and Wingard 1987; Waldron 1995). Moreover, because they live longer than men, the average woman is likely to live for many years with a host of nonlethal, but nevertheless bothersome, health complaints.

What are the possible explanations for this paradox in women's health status? Why do women currently have a mortality advantage and morbidity disadvantage? It turns out that health researchers have a good explanation for the sex differentials in mortality. These differences are primarily the result of biology, risk exposure, and health care utilization (Verbrugge 1985; Verbrugge 1990; Verbrugge and Wingard 1987; Waldron 1995). At all ages, contemporary females have a biological advantage over their male counterparts due to some combination of hormonal and genetic factors. For example, two of the three leading causes of death for both men and women—heart disease and cerebrovascular disease—develop in men at younger ages than in women, in part, because men are hormonally and genetically more vulnerable (and, women are hormonally and genetically more impervious). With respect to risk exposure, men engage in more potentially life-threatening behavior (e.g., heavy drinking, illegal drug use, reckless driving, and physical violence) and are more likely to be employed in hazardous occupations (e.g., heavy industrial and agricultural work). Finally, men are less likely than women to receive routine health care and, therefore, less likely to receive preventive care or have serious illnesses identified and treated at early stages. Collectively, these biological and cultural reasons account for women's morality advantage over men.

Whereas health researchers have a clear, albeit complex, account of observed sex differentials in mortality, the reasons for women's higher rates of sickness, pain, and disability remain, according to Lois Verbrugge (1990: 64), a "real mystery." No coherent explanations exist for women's pronounced morbidity, but rather a collection of wide-ranging and often competing interpretations. There is not even agreement, for example, about whether women really have more sickness, pain, and disability than men at all. What we know is that women are more likely to perceive themselves as ill, evaluate their illness as serious, and seek health care in response (Anson et al. 1991; Hibbard and Pope 1983; Hibbard and Pope 1986; Mirowsky and Ross 1995). In sum, at the level of perception, evaluation, and response, women *appear* to be sicker than men. Still, we simply do not know how much of this observed variation is the result of objective differences in the well-being of women and men versus subjective differences in the way they perceive, evaluate, and respond to sickness. Unlike mortality, which is an unambiguous outcome, morbidity rates necessarily capture individual judgment and assessment. Consequently, we are left with empirical facts, namely, that women report higher rates of sickness, pain, and dysfunction than men, which are unyielding to scientific certainty and open to interpretation.

It seems plausible that some of the sex differential in morbidity is more than merely perceptional and has a biological basis. Yet, women's excess in morbidity takes so many different forms that it is difficult to advance coherent biological explanations. Women suffer in far greater numbers than men from so many different types of nonfatal conditions, and these conditions are so varied in character, that developing even a series of discrete, but logically consistent, biological accounts for observed differences seems unworkable (Verbrugge 1985; Verbrugge 1990). All told, the pronounced degree and variation of women's morbidity suggest the need to think beyond "first-order" biological sex differences.To that end, some researchers suggest the sex effect on morbidity is secondary or indirect. For example, the nature of women's reproductive bodies (e.g., menstruation, pregnancies, lactation) results in their greater somatic attentiveness. Freudian informed scholars offer a variant of this thesis by asserting that a subconscious synthesis of biological differences and cultural traditions set up psychosexual developmental tasks for women that predispose them toward somatic expression (Mitchell 1975).

In addition to these explanations of the secondary role of biological sex differences, many researchers suggest the need to focus on the social and cultural reasons for the observed differences in morbidity. To what extent are the observed differences the result of gender rather than (or in addition to) sex? An implicit (and sometimes explicit) assumption advanced by women's health researchers is that various aspects of gender inequality come to be *embodied* in terms of both objective symptoms and subjective illness behavior (Bird and Rieker 1999; Ruzek et al. 1997).

With respect to the objective embodiment of gender inequality, some researchers focus on the ways women's occupational and domestic lives erode their well-being. Women's concentration in feminized, low-wage, and low-status work directly and indirectly exposes them to health risks and stresses over which they have little or no control (Bartley et al. 1992; Doyal 1995; Faucett 1997; Frankenhaeuser et al. 1991; Olsen 1997). For instance, women workers are concentrated in jobs that are sedentary and entail repetitive and routine tasks, all of which have negative health consequences (Strazdins and Bammer 2004). Women's care-giving and emotional work, both paid and unpaid, frequently requires them to deny their own physical and emotional needs to ill effect (Graham 1993; Hochschild 1983; Oakley 1993). Women's disproportionate responsibility for unpaid domestic labor, in conjunction with their paid employment, also takes a more general toll in terms of physical and emotion strain (Hochschild 1990). What is more, women's concentration in low-paying jobs can make them dependent on male partners and, in turn, more vulnerable to forces in the domestic sphere that can undermine their health. When women are subordinate economically, they are less able to make demands on partners to share in domestic labor and can be more vulnerable to physical, emotional, and sexual abuse. Women's overrepresentation among those living in poverty is also said to undermine their physical and mental health status (Reutter et al. 1998). On the other hand, the high rate of illness among particularly ambitious and successful women throughout history illustrates the potentially deleterious physical and mental health effects of challenging feminine ideals and succeeding in male-dominated fields (Silverstein and Perlick 1995).

Other researchers direct our attention to the gendered character of illness behavior and its relationship to women's high rates of morbidity (Hibbard and Pope 1983; Mechanic 1992). Some, for example, emphasize the role of gender socialization and gender ideology in accounting for sex differences in morbidity. For instance there is a better cultural fit between notions of "femininity" and "sickness" (versus "masculinity" and "sickness"), a greater willingness on the part of women to adopt the sick role, and a greater willingness on the part of physicians to endorse the sick role in their interactions with women patients (Lorber 1997). Other research highlights how women's role as guardians of family health translates into their own heightened health concern and awareness.

Of course, the way these aspects of women's lives influence their health is far from uniform. Significant mortality and morbidity disparities exist among women, most significantly in terms of class and race or ethnicity, and these health disparities reveal further negative health effects of social inequality. For example, there is a strong negative effect of class privilege on the incidence of physical morbidity and affective disorders among women (Popay et al. 1993). Black women, independent of socioeconomic position, "experience excessive levels of chronic morbidity and disability" (Geronimus 2001: 133). These class and racial differences complicate the picture considerably when taking into account the effects of gender on health.

This is by no means an exhaustive account; collectively, however, the research on women's health reveals that, beyond biological differences, women's distinctive roles (and often secondary status) in the public and private spheres (which reinforce one another) have a host of negative consequences on their well-being. Although not uniformly so, structural inequality between men and women, and supporting social practices, identities, and ideologies, are all said to contribute to the observed sex differences in morbidity.

The question of female physical and mental frailty, now more innocuously called "morbidity," has been under consideration at least since the time of Aristotle. As such, we might be wise to regard it as something of an unresolved debate. Because of some combination of objective and subjective factors, women perceive themselves as ill, evaluate their illnesses as serious, and, in response, secure health care in significantly greater numbers than do men. The exact combination of objective and subjective factors resulting in these differences is unknown, and very possibly unknowable. It may never be possible to know if women are sicker in effect or in affect (or both). Moreover, our biological bodies, as male and female, and our social lives, as men and women, are in a constant dialectical relationship to one another, making it impossible to determine to what extent the observed morbidity differences are biologically or culturally based.

As this has been a topic of intense debate for millennia, it is not the intent of this project to declare the truth about the basis of women's propensities to sickness. Rather, the focus is much less ambitious and starts with what is known and knowable. Relative to men, women are markedly *somatic*. Or, rather, relative to women, men are somatically repressed. Or, more precisely yet, the particular ways in which women are somatic show up in the social field of medicine (perhaps men's somatic tendencies show up in alternative social fields—a topic worthy of separate investigation). Women's somaticism, regardless of it causes, is a central starting point in the FMS story and, indeed, the story of women and biomedicine historically.

An Unhappy Marriage: Women and Biomedicine

In the late nineteenth century, the coming together of women patients with broadly felt embodied distresses and the nascent institution of biomedicine gave birth to the diagnostic classifications of hysteria and neurasthenia. One of the founders of neurology, Jean-Martin Charcot (1825–1893), defined hysteria as a disorder of the central nervous system, likely hereditary in nature, but his efforts to study and treat hysteric "fits" in strictly neurological terms never became part of medical orthodoxy (Goetz et al. 1995; Micale 1995). Similarly, George Beard, the American neurologists who popularized the closely related diagnosis of neurasthenia in the 1870s, considered the condition to be an organic nervous disorder triggered by excess intellectual, sexual, or digestive activity, but the organic basis of the disorder was never substantiated (Abbey and Garfinkel 1991; Ware and Kleinman 1992). Instead, by the end of the nineteenth century, physicians considered the hysteric, along with her closely related sister, the neurasthenic, to be a woman plagued by a wide range of somatic complaints of psychoneurotic origin (Micale 1995; Showalter 1997).[7] The disorders, which were poorly understood, were treated with a collection of less than efficacious therapies, including ovarian compression belts, psychoanalysis, hypnosis, and the "rest cure," which involved the avoidance of all physical and intellectual strain for several weeks, or months.

The general symptomatic and epidemiological similarities between hysteria, neurasthenia, chronic fatigue, and fibromyalgia are well documented (Abbey and Garfinkel 1991; Aronowitz 1998; Shorter 1992; Wessley 1994). In brief, with the exception of Charcot's hysterics, who suffered from dramatic seizures, the common symptoms of hysteria and neurasthenia, like those of CFS and FMS, included pain, fatigue, headaches, cognitive and mood impairments, upper respiratory symptoms, and sleep and bowel irregularities. This is a very modest list, as Beard himself noted seventy-five neurasthenic symptoms (Abbey and Garfinkel 1991). Also, as with CFS and FMS, women significantly outnumbered men among those diagnosed with these antiquated disorders, although there were proportionally more men with a diagnosis of neurasthenia than hysteria.

Whereas each of these disorders has a unique trajectory tied to its specific historical location and the medical specialty with which it is most closely associated, their similarities as categories of medical knowledge and patient experience are considerable. Among other similarities, the emergence of each of these diagnoses involves women clinically presenting common, distressing and ill-defined symptoms and physicians using their available medical knowledge and techniques to offer them imperfect explanations of, and even more imperfect remedies for, their distress.

These diagnoses, thus, demarcate a hundred-year period during which women, and certain women in particular,[8] sought biomedical explanations for distressing symptoms, which have been found less than fully intelligible in orthodox biomedical terms. Instead, for more than one hundred years, these disorders have been identified as psychosomatic and labeled with one of many vaguely specified *functional* disorders, which are conditions not linked to any known *organic* cause. From hysteria and neurasthenia to the host of contemporary functional somatic syndromes (including fibromyalgia, CFS, multiple chemical sensitivity, temporomandibular joint dysfunction syndrome, and interstitial cystitis), women sufferers fully or significantly predominate. In short, women have historically filled and still fill the ranks of contested diagnoses that grant them neither the full legitimacy of disease nor a meaningful remedy toward health.

The nature of women's somatic distress is complex, which is not to say that it is psychogenic, but when biomedicine attempts to explain it, it must do so using the same technical tools used to account for illnesses that have an identifiable, endogenous, etiological agent, or anatomical pathology. The consequences of bringing together women's complex somaticism and the biomedical perspective are addressed in Kaja Finkler's (1994) book *Women in Pain: Gender and Morbidity in Mexico*. Specifically, Finkler contends that women suffer from so many nonfatal illnesses of unknown origin because so many different types of social and interpersonal adversities—"life's lesions"—negatively impact their well-being, yet such lesions elude the medical gaze. The mismatch between the factors that give rise and meaning to women's somatic tendencies and the orientation and methods of biomedicine must be considered as a possible explanation for why women fill the ranks of a host of past and present-day contested illnesses. The diagnostic making of FMS and its continued contested status suggest the plausibility of just such an explanation, returning us to the puzzle set out at the outset of this chapter: the *present absence* of sex and gender from FMS.

Rheumatology, the Woman Problem, and the Feminized Idiom of Tender Points

Smythe makes no mention of an association between fibrositis and women in either the 1972 or 1979 chapter in *Arthritis and Allied Conditions*. Moreover, in a seminal article he published with co-researcher Harvey Moldofsky in 1977, the sex of "ten fibrositis patients" is unspecified (1977: 929). Interestingly, Smythe and Moldofsky open the article with two Biblical quotes from Job, a frequently referenced FMS sufferer, giving the disorder a decidedly male face. In addition, they present a medical illustration (Figure 2.1) displaying the location of tender points, using both a male and female figure, an illustration Smythe incorporated in *Arthritis and Allied Conditions* in 1979.[9]

Notwithstanding this early surface neutrality, the diagnostic entrepreneurs were well aware that their patients with FMS were principally women. Objectively, their clinical research during the 1980s revealed the overwhelming feminization of the disorder. In some of their clinical research, in fact, patients with FMS were *all* women. In the American College of Rheumatology (ACR) study, the figure was approximately 90 percent. Their diagnostic research is also peppered with descriptions of the typical patient with FMS, demonstrating their recognition that sufferers were primarily women and that their complaints fit into the context of their

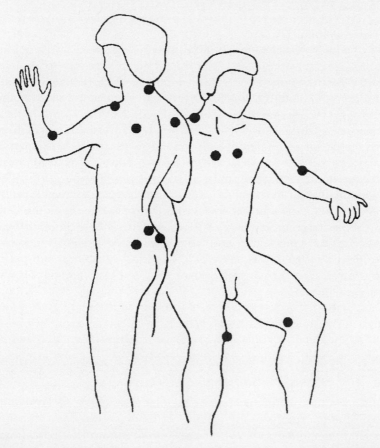

Figure 2.1   Tender Points in Fibrositis. Hugh Smythe and Harvey Moldofsky, 1977. "Two contributions to understanding of the 'fibrositis' syndrome." *Bulletin on the Rheumatic Diseases* 28: 928–931.

lives as women. For example, the following is a case vignette from a landmark diagnostic study that reads much like Betty Friedan's (1963) description of "the problem that has no name" from *The Feminine Mystique:*[10]

A 30-yr-old, white female presented with "aches all over," especially in low back, upper gluteal regions, neck, shoulders and hands, for the past 10 yr. She also complained of stiffness in the morning and evening. In general, her symptoms were aggravated by inactivity, damp and cold weather, mental stress and excess physical activities, and relived by warm weather, moderate activities and a hot bath. She felt tired and over-worked as a housewife, and admitted that she was a somewhat anxious person. . . . Physical examination showed completely normal joint findings. . . . All laboratory tests . . . were normal. Treatment included reassurance regarding the benign nature of primary fibromyalgia, salicylate therapy for pain, and Elavil 25 mg at bedtime for better sleep (Yunus et al. 1981: 156–57).

This vignette is a powerful example of the medical framing of women's common and broadly felt somatic distresses. As the patient is described, something is both very wrong and not wrong at all: the experience of aches and pains, exhaustion, overwork, and anxiety is met with an altogether normal physical examination and laboratory results. The remedy—a hot bath, reassurance, aspirin, and antidepressants—is, at once, inexact and benevolently condescending. The aim is not, however, to highlight the potentially patronizing character of the male doctor-female patient dynamic. Rather, the crucial point is that diagnostic entrepreneurs, such as the ones referenced above, were struggling, in earnest, to frame women's distress medically within the conceptual category of FMS. Indeed, the very idea of FMS, itself, is an attempt on the part of the diagnostic entrepreneurs to organize women's common complaints within a biomedical model.

The basis of this argument starts with women's heightened somatic tendencies in general and the expression of pain as one particular way those tendencies manifest themselves. Musculoskeletal pain, already among the most common symptoms reported in the general public, is significantly more common among women than men (Barsky and Borus 1999; Fillingim 2000). A 1999 Gallup survey found that nearly half of all American women experience pain on a daily basis (Arthritis Foundation 2003). The report of pain in multiple anatomic sites also is significantly more common among women than it is among men. Moreover, women are far more likely to evaluate their pain as intense and 50 percent more likely to have had pain-related absences from work (Arthritis Foundation 2003). Not surprisingly, therefore, women have higher utilization rates for pain-related health care (Unruh 1996). In sum, compared with men, women are more likely clinically to report troublesome, chronic, widespread pain, which is why the diagnostic entrepreneurs found themselves grappling with such a large residual pool of women patients in the first place.

But the large group of women patients that the entrepreneurs faced reported not only pain but also many additional distressing and seemingly disconnected symptoms, all lacking an established pathophysiology. The only available diagnosis for such patients within existing rheumatological nomenclature—psychogenic rheumatism—medically marginalized patients and their complaints and, by extension, professionally marginalized those who, out of interest or necessity, studied and treated such patients. Moreover, the conflation of women and the presentation of multiple, unexplainable symptoms only further discredited patients and their experiences and devalued the work of their attendant clinician researchers.

The task facing the diagnostic entrepreneurs was not to describe, explain, or resolve the drudgery of housewifery briefly noted in the above case vignette or the often omnipresent and multifaceted corrosive effects of gender inequality on women's general physical and mental well-being. Such tasks are not a part of biomedicine's orientation nor do they fall within its jurisdictional authority. Rather, as summarized by Peter Freund and colleagues (2003: 220–22), some of the orienting assumptions of the biomedical model include a clear divide between mind and body and the corresponding presumption that physical disease can be measured in the form of disordered bodily processes. Moreover, the metaphor of the *body as machine* (i.e., various parts of the body function in the state of health and malfunction in the state of disease) encourages biomedicine to divide the body into parts that can be studied and treated in isolation of the whole—a trend augmented by medical specialization that declares expertise over one body part or body system. The biomedical body is both disconnected from its social context and further partitioned and atomized at the sub-organism level. Biomedicine, in sum, is conceptually oriented toward finding and treating discrete pathology in the parts or systems of the individual body.

As such, the professional task facing the diagnostic entrepreneurs was to determine if women patients' broadly felt subjective distresses, *whatever* their origins or however complex, could be organized within the boundaries of evidence-based medicine, generally, and within the sphere of rheumatological authority, specifically. At issue was whether some measurement of musculoskeletal embodiment that systematically accompanied women patients' subjective reports could be used to extricate a subset of them from the residual category of psychogenic rheumatism. In sum, could they translate women patients' wide-ranging subjective suffering into biomedical language over which they had jurisdictional authority? We know from Chapter 1 that the answer to this question is yes.

From Smythe onward, the idea crystallized that the broad and mundane constellation of FMS symptoms could be given clinical representation through the presence of tenderness in characteristic locations. The ACR criteria formalized the idea: FMS is characterized by pain in all four quadrants of the body and tenderness in 11 of 18 tender points. The essentially tautological construction of these criteria was described in Chapter 1. As noted there, the diagnostic entrepreneurs defined patients with FMS by the presence of the multiple tender points and then, unsurprisingly, found that multiple tender points best distinguished patients from controls. But the FMS tautology is also *gendered*. The diagnostic entrepreneurs started with women's general somatic distress and ended up by embedding measurements of women's general somatic distress in the FMS diagnostic criteria.

As case in point, not only are women more likely than men to report chronic widespread pain and pain in multiple anatomic sites, but positive tender points are significantly more common in women than in men. On this score, the evidence is clear: At all ages, women report more positive tender points than men and less pressure is required to evoke tenderness at tender point locations in women than men (Wolfe et al. 1995a; Wolfe and Cathey 1985; Yunus et al. 2000). In addition, the sex discrepancy in number of positive tender points exists irrespective of underlying disease. In others words, healthy women have more positive tender points than healthy men, and women diagnosed with FMS have more positive tender points than men diagnosed with FMS (Wolfe and Cathey 1985; Wolfe et al. 1995b). In a nonclinical population, Frederick Wolfe and coworkers (1995a) found women were ten times more likely to have the required eleven tender points necessary to meet the ACR criteria than were men. Whatever tender points might or might not be organically speaking, they appear to be a highly feminized idiom of distress.

Consequently, both of the subjectively based criteria at the heart of the ACR definition (widespread pain and multiple tender points) are endemic among women. In purely practical terms, the feminization of the disorder was conceptually and tautologically assured. The diagnostic entrepreneurs started with a common feminized mode of somatic expression and the existing criteria assure that most of those diagnosed with FMS will be women.

But, while the diagnostic entrepreneurs created FMS principally from the suffering of women patients, nevertheless some men were in some of their diagnostic studies. In the ACR study, for instance, nearly 10 percent of the patients were men, and, in line with good technical practices, the entrepreneurs sex-matched patients and controls (i.e., nearly 10 percent of the controls were also men). In terms of research design, sex was a "control" variable. Controlling for sex, the diagnostic entrepreneurs then used statistical tests to measure all variety of between-group differences, thereby specifying the characteristics that distinguished between patients and controls. Logically, however, sex could not possibly distinguish between patients and controls, because the two groups had been sex-matched at the outset, nor could other observable differences between patients and controls be the indirect result of sex differences. In line with this logic, the criterial studies, including that of the ACR, conceptually implied that the FMS diagnostic criteria were uniformly salient, irrespective of sex.

Controlling for sex is a common practice in biomedical research. Generally, however, this practice construes sex as an "irritant" variable (Taylor 1997, quoted in Rieker and Bird 2000: 101). Rarely do researchers systematically investigate within-group differences or test for interaction effects (Rieker and Bird 2000: 101). This was the case in FMS diagnostic research. Although the research design of the ACR study implies the uniformity of diagnostic criteria for women and men, the study does not explicitly address whether this is indeed the case. The ACR study does not address the sensitivity, specificity, or accuracy of its criteria for women versus men. Rather, the logic of their study restricted their focus to what were considered to be sex-independent similarities among those with FMS, and so, at a conceptual level, skirted the disorder's overwhelming feminization. As a result, the study failed to address whether the criteria overdiagnosed the conditions of women and underdiagnosed those of men.

Thus, on one hand, FMS represents an attempt on the part of rheumatologists to organize and understand women's somatic suffering within a biomedical model. Through a series of internal analogies, technological processes, and statistical procedures, the diagnostic entrepreneurs were able to translate a vast and disparate cluster of women's somatic complaints into an embodied measurement. Simply put, FMS criteria are a template that captures women's general somaticism. Yet, on the other hand, the specific practices used by rheumatologists in this undertaking conceptually obscured the gendered character of the FMS construction. The ACR criteria possess the allure of sex and gender neutrality when, in fact, they are a proxy or technical surrogate for women's embodied distress. Being a woman is nearly necessary, although clearly not sufficient, for being diagnosed with FMS, and yet this fact was written out of FMS at the diagnostic level. Even as the practical knowledge of FMS fully recognizes its feminization (i.e., clinician researchers know that FMS is highly feminized), the codified knowledge of FMS is abstracted from this reality.

The point here is not to suggest that the diagnostic entrepreneurs were foolish or cunning for including so few men in their studies (or for including any of them at all, given their small numbers). Presumably, the female-male ratio of their research subjects is an approximate reflection of the female-male ratio of clinical FMS populations. The diagnostic entrepreneurs conceptually obscured the gendered character of the FMS construction, not because they *deviated* from standard medical practice, but indeed because of their *adherence* to it. They uncritically applied a widely used research design: They sex-matched patients and controls but failed to assess (or report) what, if any, sex variability was couched therein.

In sum, they followed the common practice by treating sex as an irritant variable. This was true in the ACR criteria study and continues to be protocol in most FMS research. It is also worth noting that oversampling for men with FMS at a rate that would allow for valid sex subgroup analyses would have been costly in terms of both time and money (Satel 2000).

Nevertheless, what remains puzzling is that, despite the overwhelming feminization of FMS, clinician researchers have not asked themselves, "I wonder why so many women have FMS?" Nor have they asked themselves, "I wonder if our FMS criteria are themselves sex biased?" It is precisely the failure to address such questions that I have called the "present absence" of sex and gender from the idea of FMS. This term focuses our attention on the fact that, even as everyone engaged in this research is well aware of the feminization of the disorder, almost no one has explicitly addressed this reality. Most importantly, what results is a body of knowledge about FMS that skirts sex and gender at the conceptual level. This is seen in the ACR criteria themselves and in the substantive agenda of research primarily focused on the role of sex-neutral neurobiological abnormalities, muscle pathology, and psychopathology in the etiology of FMS.

The present absence of sex and gender is largely the result of biomedicine's endogenous orientation, the specific technoscientific practices used in clinical diagnostic research, and rheumatology's traditional jurisdictional focus on musculoskeletal pain. In addition, however, it did not hurt rheumatologists, professionally speaking, to skirt the overwhelming feminization of the disorder to avoid the awkwardness of dealing with the combination of women patients and unexplained illness. Jurisdictional expansion, through the creation of a new diagnosis, is dependent on defining, in abstract terms, biomedicine's authority over a particular problem (Abbott 1988). Simply noting the many women with a host of unexplainable physical and emotional symptoms would have been insufficiently abstract to make a new jurisdictional claim. Although the diagnostic entrepreneurs may never have attempted to hide the feminization of FMS, neither did their analytic focus call attention to it. Defining FMS as a chronic pain disorder characterized by multiple tender points offered them a way to approach women's somatic distress in a nominally non-gendered, biomedical language—an important tool in further distancing FMS from its immediate predecessor, psychogenic rheumatism.

Finally, the diagnostic entrepreneurs found approaching women's somatic symptoms from a narrow biological perspective a suitable strategy for negotiating the cultural demands of "political correctness."[11] As a result of broad political and cultural changes associated with the women's movement and specific transformations in health care in the wake of the women's health movement, it is no longer possible for biomedicine simply to dismiss women's complaints as hysterical. Nevertheless, finding a way to address women's overrepresentation among those with medically unexplainable symptoms and contested illnesses remains problematic. One leading FMS researcher spoke directly and frankly to me on this point: "You run into problems doing this kind of work. Women are more prone to psychosomatic illness. We avoid problems in part by approaching these things biologically." Thus, in the context of raised feminist cultural consciousness, one paradoxical trend within biomedicine (as seen in the diagnostic making of FMS) is a hyperbiological approach to women's unexplainable complaints, which ultimately accelerates the tendency toward medicalization of their distress.

In sum, as the constraints of political correctness, or "PC," culture trickle down into the institution of medicine, they intersect with biomedicine's longstanding propensity to frame women's normal embodiment as pathological, and combine to encourage the medicalization of women's somatic distress. FMS takes common feminized expressions of distress and frames them as aberrant. However, because those expressions represent a very general feminized idiom of suffering, FMS is an *immense* conceptual category under which many different forms of distress can be housed. This tendency became even more pronounced with increased flexibility in the FMS criteria proposed in the *Copenhagen Declaration*. Consequently, a wide range of women's distress is now readily medicalized under FMS, but for many of the reasons discussed above, it is a *contested* medicalization. FMS is a condition whose organic basis is questioned by many biomedical clinicians, but to which a biomedical diagnosis is nevertheless routinely applied, thereby stranding millions of women diagnosed with the disorder to cope with their somatic distress without the cultural support and legitimization that a diagnosis ordinarily brings.

3

Similar-but-Different: The Fibromyalgia Syndrome Illness Experience

T hus far, we have discussed the idea of fibromyalgia syndrome (FMS) as biomedical knowledge, but now we turn our attention the experience of those living with FMS. This is the first of several chapters devoted to describing the subjective experience of FMS, based on interviews with thirty women diagnosed with the disorder.[1] All thirty women are white, one is Hispanic; they range in age from twenty-eight to sixty-five years with a mean age of forty-eight years; and they have an average educational level of approximately thirteen years. In each of these regards, this sample compares closely with that found in community prevalence studies. This is not to suggest that this small sample is representative of those who suffer from FMS in general. However, in terms of a few key demographic factors (race or ethnicity, age, and education), this sample does not appear to be markedly dissimilar from what we know about those who suffer from FMS in published population studies (White et al. 1999; Wolfe et al. 1995).[2] The focus of this study, however, is markedly different from epidemiological or clinical research on FMS. The question posed here is what can we learn from listening to the FMS stories of thirty women who suffer from FMS?

The first thing we can learn is that there is a shared chronicle of FMS.[3] For example, one need only speak to a few sufferers to come away with a clear appreciation of the devastating impact of FMS. In the face of an overwhelming set of symptoms, tasks that were once effortless and routine become unimaginably difficult or, indeed, impossible. Plans and dreams for the future become derailed or abandoned. Some sufferers become, and remain, disabled, whereas most others move in and out of periods of disablement, called "flares" or "flare-ups." Instead of dividing one's energies among the component pieces that constitute a full life, the daily existence of a person who suffers from FMS is often totally absorbed by the management of chronic symptoms and the avoidance of consuming flares. The impact of overwhelming and changeable symptoms on the lives of those who suffer from FMS is explored in greater depth in Chapter 4.

Another essential feature of FMS described by the women in this study is the burden of routinely having their illness called into question by both medical professionals and the lay public. Before having their condition diagnosed as FMS, the women spent an average of six and a half years going from doctor to doctor in search of an explanation for their intense symptoms. The symptoms alone can be physically and emotionally distressing, but the response of disbelief on the part of the medical and lay public further increases sufferers' social isolation and dark mood. It is for this reason that the women in this study emphasize their struggle for a diagnosis and the profound sense of relief and validation that accompanied finally being diagnosed of FMS, even in the absence of promising therapeutics. These other shared aspects of FMS—the prolonged search for a diagnosis and the importance of learning of one—are the focus of Chapters 5 and 6, respectively.

Yet, despite the impression of the regularity to FMS, based on these and other noteworthy similarities, the details surrounding each woman's illness also reveal their marked dissimilarities. They have different symptom composites, divergent consequences that brought them to near or total disablement, variable levels of everyday functioning, and disparate responses to similar treatments. Even as women's accounts of their illness share a common plot—organized around the devastating consequences of a set of unexplainable symptoms and the importance of their eventual diagnosis—the specific details of their illnesses are distinct.

For example, women describe considerable overlap in their symptoms but no uniform set of symptoms is found among them. Although diagnostically necessary, pain holds a different position within the symptom composites of different sufferers. Pain is unambiguously Mary's primary symptom; however, depression and pain are equal players in Alice's illness; and Doris finds the combination of fatigue, depression, and memory loss far more debilitating than the pain. What is more, the extensive list of possible FMS symptoms makes the number of permutations vast. In addition to pain, fatigue, and depression, Phyllis cannot breath and her heart races; Wendy has bladder and yeast infections, vision abnormalities, "fibrofog," and chemical sensitivity; and Robin experiences seizures and chronic dizziness. In fact, the confusion associated with multiple permutations of related FMS symptoms resulted in the American College of Rheumatology's final decision to exclude them as possible criteria altogether (Wolfe et al. 1990). Ultimately, one can candidly state that there are nearly as many FMS symptom composites as there are those who suffer from FMS.

The most striking variation among the women's FMS experiences is found in the descriptions of their illness onset. Mary became ill in her late fifties, concurrent with a work-related, repetitive strain injury. Hannah's symptoms started in her mid forties, in conjunction with menopause. Valerie's illness progressed during her twenties and thirties, interwoven with difficult pregnancies and the death of her husband. Suzanne became suddenly ill after a flulike sickness in her mid twenties. Emily's symptoms came about when she was a teenager and active in high school athletics. Phyllis describes anxiety and pain dating back to childhood, but her symptoms intensified in her twenties, a time during which her husband abused her physically on a daily basis. Paula traces her FMS to a serious neck injury sustained as a teenager, and Ellen reports that her FMS might be connected to a traumatic event she witnessed when she was less than a year old.

As can be seen, both the age at which a woman became ill and the constellation of events leading up to her illness diverge widely. For many, physical or emotional trauma (e.g., a serious injury, surgery, death of a loved one) is closely timed with the onset of the illness, whereas, for others, a common illness or physical change (e.g., the flu, pregnancy, menopause) corresponds to illness onset. For still others, no trigger or precipitating experience can be identified; they simply became and remained ill. Some did so quickly, whereas others did so gradually over a long period of time. As with others who suffer from FMS who have been described in published medical research, the women in this study reveal little uniformity in terms of "risk factors" contributing to their illness onset (Hawley and Wolfe 2000). As such, providing a conceptually coherent biomedical explanation linking these widely divergent patterns in illness onset is highly problematic.

The women also differ in terms of their illness course or prognosis. For Barbara, Emily, and Courtney, their symptoms of FMS became more bearable and less intense over time. This contrasts with a progression in symptom severity for Wendy, Phyllis, and Sally. Similarly, although all of the women describe their symptoms as debilitating, their levels of daily functioning differ radically. In general, the women fall in between the extremes of Karen, who works four days a week as a bookkeeper and does much of the daily housework for her husband and sons, and Robin, who has not left her house in eight months and rarely manages to leave her bed. Neither Karen nor Robin represents the average level of functioning of those living with FMS, either in this study or in studies in the medical literature (Henriksson and Burckhardt 1996; Ledingham et al. 1993). That said, it is hard to say what the "average" level of functioning might be. Not only does functionality vary greatly from person to person, but it also varies dramatically as any one person moves in and out of flare-ups.

Finally, the women also have very dissimilar responses to similar therapeutic interventions, even as none of them describes their FMS treatment as particularly effective. Hannah's condition, as with many others in this study, improved appreciably with the use of pain medications and antidepressants, whereas Phyllis, Robin, and Alice experienced insignificant improvements in response to the same regimen. Betsy wildly praises the same biofeedback technique that magnifies Jessica's migraines. Procaine (Novocain) injections into painful joints left Cindy severely bruised and unable to move for weeks, but Emily is grateful to receive them every three months. Courtney and Barbara insist on struggling through light daily exercise as a way of preserving their limited mobility, whereas exercise of any sort dramatically worsens Karen and Wendy's pain and fatigue. Likewise, acupuncture temporarily alleviates the pain for some, but elevates it for others; massage therapy is rated as effective and ineffective in equal measure; and "body work" treatments (e.g., cranial sacral therapy) are both touted and dismissed. Although anecdotal, the treatment experiences of these women parallel findings in the published treatment research. To date, orthodox and alternative treatments of FMS have been unremarkable and inconsistent (Carrette 1995; Goldenberg 1999; Wolfe et al. 1997a). Moreover, the treatment modalities that have illustrated some limited efficacy (pain medications, antidepressants, exercise, and cognitive or behavioral interventions) are "nonspecific;" that is, they are also effective in the treatment of any of a large number of other conditions (Makela 1999; Goldenberg et al. 2004).

In sum, and in line with findings from much larger clinical and community studies, the women in this study have different (1) combinations of symptoms, (2) symptom onsets, (3) exposure to "risk factors," and (4) prognoses and responses to treatment. No orthodox epidemiological concept links those who suffer from FMS and, consequently, many argue that there is no empirical support for FMS as a distinct biomedical entity with a coherent natural history (Gran 2003; Makela 1999). Nevertheless, women's descriptions of FMS do have a core regularity that is powerfully evident. Certainly, sufferers understand themselves as being engaged in a common struggle against their shared illness and social prejudice—an understanding palpably revealed by visiting any in-person or Internet FMS support group.

One, thus, is left with thirty accounts of FMS that sound remarkably similar and yet hardly alike. The striking similarities in the descriptions of FMS provided by the women in this study offer compelling evidence of the disorder's authenticity. Yet, at the same time that women affirm the shared character of FMS, each woman's unique story of illness portends the difficulties of organizing their disparate experiences within a unified disease model. From a biomedical perspective, the absence of a coherent natural history raises questions about the diagnostic legitimacy of FMS, but from a sociological perspective the similar-yet-different quality of FMS raises interesting questions inviting further investigation. Minimally, the unmistakable uniformity with which women describe their FMS corroborates its existence, if not as a disease, then as an illness experience. This argument will be developed in great detail over the course of the next several chapters, but first it is necessary to introduce some of the conceptual tools that will be used in this endeavor. In particular, a few words are necessary about the general *illness experience* literature and its reliance on the key concept of *illness narratives*.

The Illness Experience

In pre- and early industrial times, infectious diseases (e.g., tuberculosis, influenza, cholera), were a frequent cause of death. Epidemics were commonplace, infant mortality rate was high, and life expectancy was low. In our developed or postindustrial U.S. society, by contrast, we face few fears of deadly infectious disease; infant mortality rate is low, and life expectancy has reached nearly seventy-seven years.[4] These dramatic demographic shifts are the result of large-scale political and economic changes that have significantly improved the average citizen's standard of living and, to a lesser extent, life-extending medical technologies (McKinlay and McKinlay 2001). With the benefits of our expanding life span, however, have come new problems and concerns. For example, although most of us can now expect to live well into late adulthood, most of us can also expect to live for years, or even decades, with at least one chronic illness and its corresponding restrictions.

In response to these significant trends in mortality and morbidity, medical sociologists have turned their attention to describing how individuals live *with* chronic illness. Peter Conrad (1987) was among the first to suggest such a line of inquiry, but other sociologists and social scientists were quick to follow. Among the central questions Conrad and others pose: How do the chronically ill understand and make sense of their illness? How do they adapt to, and cope with, the biological and social restrictions of chronic illness? And, how do they deflect self-erosion in the face of those biological and social restrictions? These are questions asked by researchers interested in the *illness experience.*

As these questions reveal, the theoretical and empirical focus of illness experience research is the subjective experience of symptoms rather than the objective nature of disease. As such, among the intellectual roots guiding this research are the insights provided by a phenomenological approach to the sociology of everyday life. Simply stated, phenomenology is the study of how people experience everyday life and the way in which they instill their everyday life with meaning.[5] Health scholars make use of phenomenology, and the work of sociologist Alfred Schutz (1899–1959) in particular, to investigate how people experience illness—or the lived experience of symptoms—and the meaning illness has in their lives.[6] This field of study describes the impact of symptoms on what phenomenologists refer to as the individual's "life world."

An individual's life world is his or her ready-at-hand framework for making sense of the world (Schutz 1967: 133). As a concept, life world directs our attention to the taken-for-granted or common sense thinking about reality. This everyday human consciousness is fittingly called "the natural attitude" because it is the familiar, routine, seemingly natural way of being. We move through our everyday lives, going about our everyday affairs, constantly drawing on these everyday assumptions, but we do so in ways that are not fully conscious to us and about which we suspend doubt.[7] At least, such is the case until something happens to disrupt our taken-for-granted reality. In other words, the natural attitude of everyday life exists as an experiential foundation "until further notice" (Berger and Luckmann 1967: 24). For a host of reasons, chronic illness represents a moment when notice is given—an instant when the taken-for-grantedness of everyday life becomes destabilized.

Any serious or chronic illness leads to a breakdown of the normal experience of self and of self in relation to others. Our sense of who we are is fundamentally linked to the routine functioning of our bodies. Our body, in effect, moves us out into the world of social interactions and performances through which we come to constitute our sense of self (Berger and Luckmann 1967; Goffman 1961). When serious illness limits our mobility, it limits personal and work performances, which, in turn, undermines our pre-illness identity. Something of a "civil death" is associated with serious illnesses to the extent that those who are ill are restricted from the everyday social interactions and performances through which they acquire self-meaning.[8] It is for this reason that chronic illness represents a "biographical disruption"(Bury 1982).

The erosion of self and life world is even more pronounced for those suffering from illnesses that lack biomedical—and thus cultural—legitimacy. For example, because the subjective experience of chronic pain cannot be confirmed medically, chronic pain itself is denied cultural meaning and the experience of chronic pain is denied cultural legitimacy (Hilbert 1984; Morris 1991; Scarry 1985). Similarly, individuals with medically contested illnesses, such as FMS, chronic fatigue syndrome (CFS), and multiple chemical sensitive (MCS), endure the burden of experiencing their symptoms in the context of both medical and public skepticism (Aronowitz 1998; Kroll-Smith and Floyd 1997; Strauss 1994; Ware 1999; Ware and Kleinman 1992). Leslie Cooper (1997: 202), for instance, speaks of the "double disruption" of debilitating symptoms and medical disbelief that characterize myalgic encephalomyelitis (ME), the British label for CFS. In sum, individuals with illnesses that are medically marginalized have their experience of reality routinely called into question, leading to the discrediting of self and social isolation.

Yet, individuals do not merely accept the mortification of self and disruption of the life world brought on by serious illness or the dual threat of debilitating yet medically unexplainable illnesses. Instead, they labor to make sense of their illness and imbue it with meaning. Moreover, faced with uncertainty, restrictions, and losses, individuals seek to understand their illness in relation to who they have been in the past and who they can be in the future. In the process, they work to reestablish a sense of self and repair the basic parameters of everyday life. It should be obvious that performing these tasks that accompany any serious illness take on an even greater urgency for sufferers of contested illnesses.

Sociologists and other social and behavioral scientists are not alone in their commitment to understanding the illness experience, generally, or that of contested illnesses, in particular. A small number of biomedical clinician researchers are also interested in studying how individuals live with chronic illness and its meaning in their lives; their interest emerges out of necessity. Although the central and emerging challenges facing contemporary biomedicine primarily involve managing complex, chronic illnesses, its methods and treatments are typically better suited for acute illnesses where a discrete pathogen or physical dysfunction can be identified and a technical solution administered. Chronic illnesses are etiologically complex and, by definition, persistent and relatively unresponsive to quick or decisive technological fixes. Physicians and other health care providers, therefore, increasingly find themselves managing an individual's illness rather than treating their disease. Accordingly, as with social scientists, biomedical clinicians and researchers have also become interested in the subjective experience of illness in addition and in relation to the objective state of disease. In the words of anthropologist and psychiatrist Arthur Kleinman, who straddles the social science and biomedical worlds:

> Chronic illness is nothing if not various, as many-sided and differing as our lives. That is why, if we are to understand the meaning of illness, we cannot focus on the content.... Instead, we must inquire into the structure of illness meanings: the manner in which illness is made meaningful, the processes of creating meaning, and the social situations and psychological reactions that determine and are determined by the meanings (1988: 185).

Illness Narratives

Illness narratives are one way that researchers, including Kleinman, capture the methods chronically ill individuals use in their search for illness meaning (Ezzy 2000; Kugelmann 1999; Phillips 1990; Riessman 1990). Illness narratives are stories of symptoms and self that construct meaning through the sequential ordering of important life events. They are empirical examples, as it were, of illness meaning as structured by "wounded storytellers" (Frank 1995) themselves. This recent narrative turn in health research represents a partial breakdown in the long observed division of labor between social and medical researchers. Whereas medical clinicians and research scientists typically study *the natural and objective properties of disease*, scholars in the social sciences and humanities typically study *the cultural and subjective character of illness*. Yet, during the last several decades, the binaries at the heart of this division have been breached and researchers in medicine, the social sciences, and the humanities alike consider how stories individuals tell about illness provide insight into the complexity of illness as part of the human experience.

Physician Oliver Sacks has received considerable public attention for his best-selling books based on his patient's illness narratives. In the preface to *The Man Who Mistook His Wife for a Hat*, Sacks (1987: viii) recommends that biomedicine compensate for its tendency to treat the human subject primarily as a host for pathology by turning its attention to detailed clinical case histories, or narratives. Humans, according to Sacks, do not simply contract diseases; they also fall "radically into sickness." As a result, only when we listen to patient narratives "do we have a 'who' as well as a 'what,' a real person, a patient, in relation to disease" (Sacks 1987: viii). By listing to illness narratives we focus on the experience of suffering rather than the natural history of disease. Given the complexity and durability of chronic diseases that pervade contemporary society, illness narratives are an important supplement to biomedicine's strictly biological approach.

This is particularly the case for medically contested illnesses that continue to elude biomedicine and resist being easily organized within a biomedical framework. Moreover, because women are more likely than men to live with chronic illnesses, including contested chronic illnesses such as FMS, studying women's illness narratives seems a particularly germane line of inquiry in terms of bringing women's distress to the fore. Indeed, this approach intersects with feminist concerns regarding biomedicine's failure to understand women's health as emerging from the social contexts in which they live—a failure, as seen in the preceding chapter, that results in the tendency to misrepresent or medicalize women's embodied experiences. Insofar as much of the current uncertainty and conflict surrounding FMS is a consequence of a mismatch between the character of women's distress and the nature of biomedicine, exploring women's FMS illness narratives provides an opportunity to discern the complex meaning and structure of FMS in the lives of women.

Even with the lack of uniformity in the biomedical parameters and trajectory of FMS, a shared resonance is found in the narrative accounts of living with FMS, as told by the women in this study. There is, we might say, a shared *social* reality to FMS. Sociology's contribution is to study and make sense of the social reality of illness as distinct from its biomedical reality (Freidson 1971).

4

The Symptomatic Self and the Life World

Wendy: Fibromyalgia is very debilitating. I can't work anymore. It's hard to explain because there isn't any one thing you can put your finger on, but it's everything in combination. It's like a domino factor. It starts out with achy muscles and it just goes from there. If you're talking about fibromyalgia being debilitating in terms of working, you tell me who's going to hire me when I tell them that they could not depend on me. I can't handle any stress, I have no memory, I can't concentrate, I can't spell anymore. Would you want to hire me? You don't know from day to day what you're going to be like or how you're going to feel. If I had to get up every morning and get dressed and drive to a job by a certain time, the costs of doing that would be enough to send me into a flare.[1]

Wendy provides a typical description of fibromyalgia syndrome (FMS). As with others who suffer from FMS, she struggles for words to explain how the debilitating and capricious symptoms are collectively greater than the sum of their parts. Without question, the most striking similarity in women's narratives of FMS is the cumulative, destructive, and unpredictable character of their symptoms. This chapter presents a detailed account of these shared symptomatic features of FMS. In particular, it presents women's narrative accounts of FMS symptoms and the impact those symptoms have on their everyday lives. What follows is a description of how the FMS illness experience erodes the self and the taken-for-granted life world.

The FMS Symptom Composite: Greater Than the Sum of Its Parts

The symptoms of FMS have already been listed several times thus far in this book, but merely cataloging a collection of symptoms tells us little about the lived experience of those with such symptoms. One reason for this conceptual gap is that the FMS symptom inventory is largely made up of physical complaints we all experience from time to time. Pain and fatigue, for instance, are the two most common complaints for which the general public seeks medical care. Likewise, most of the associated symptoms of FMS (mood, cognitive, digestive, sleep disruptions) are also routine distresses.

We are all more or less familiar with each of the component symptoms of FMS. We have had pain in our hips, necks, backs, or joints. We have had injuries in the wake of an auto accident or bicycle mishap. We ache after a day of "overdoing it" in the garden or playing softball after a ten-year athletic hiatus. We have all found ourselves too tired to face the day, feeling so exhausted we can barely keep ourselves awake in the late afternoon, or so depleted that we take to our bed hours in advance of our routine. We have all been down, blue, overwhelmed, and anxious. On occasion, we all forget items at the grocery store, misplace our car keys, forget we put a kettle on to boil, and transpose numbers. Finally, the torments of stomach and bowel distress are regrettably common to many of us, as are sleepless and restless nights.

Although we are likely acquainted with the individual complaints of FMS, what is unfamiliar is the chronic and intense character that these otherwise routine symptoms assume as they coalesce into a devastating symptom composite. The women provide gripping descriptions of how the persistent and manifold symptoms come together to exponential effect. The symptoms build on one another until their collective result is nothing short of overwhelming. Typical examples follow.

Courtney: You have to deal with so many parts of it. First, there is the depression. There's a huge amount of depression. Of course, I have medication for that and the medicine helps hugely. The two highest things on the list you have to deal with are extreme fatigue and the pain that is everywhere in your body. And even the pain, a person learns to deal with that, but with the fatigue, you just can't get past that.

Alice: The physical hurt, and the psychological hurt, and the combination of both, is overwhelming.

Sally: It spreads and the pain level gets worse and worse and worse. You think it cannot get worse, but it gets worse. I will get so tired that I cannot even stand up and take a shower. My mind was as sharp as a steel trap, but now I cannot find words that I know. I have no memory, no concentration. I can't judge the distance between the ground and my feet. I have dizziness, anxiety. I am on antidepressants. I have IBS [irritable bowel syndrome], rheumatoid [arthritis], headaches, and pain from the top of my skull to the bottom of my toes. The bottoms of my feet feel bruised. I cannot go barefoot any more. In addition, my immune system started going nuts. I have bronchitis four to five times a year. If I get around someone with a cold, I get pneumonia. My skin burns from head to toe.

Ellen: Actually, I have quite a few of the symptoms of fibromyalgia. They are mostly physical, but there are some other symptoms that it causes: chronic pain, chronic fatigue, "crampy" muscles, numbness, light "headedness", muscle spasms, loss of balance, swelling, night sweats, headaches, redness and hot spots, ringing of the ears, chest pain, mouth pain, restlessness, itchy skin. It affects your hair. I have lack of coordination, foot pain, weakness, shaking, racing heart. It affects your memory and concentration. It can affect you in a way that can make you confused sometimes. Nausea, dizziness, heartburn, blurred vision, stomach problems.

In different ways, these four women portray the destructive character of the FMS symptom constellation. Courtney and Alice highlight the physical and psychological components of FMS as well as their combined impact. Sally and Ellen's approach, listing their multiple symptoms, one after the other, effectively conveys their cumulative weight. Because Ellen provides such a substantial list, and because she switches between phrases that describe symptoms she clearly has ("*I have* lack of coordination") and phrases that describe symptoms one could have as part of FMS ("*It* affects your memory and concentration."), I asked her to clarify her remarks. Was she describing her own symptoms or describing FMS symptoms in general? "I experience all of these symptoms and I keep track of them. I document all of them." In fact, Ellen was reading from a list she takes to doctors' appointments to make sure she mentions each of her symptoms and their variation over time. Other women also keep running lists of symptoms, a technique encouraged by FMS self-help resources for maximizing one's limited time with health care providers and offsetting the liabilities of the cognitive confusion routinely called "fibrofog." Margaret, for instance, explains her need for a symptom list: "How else could I remember so many symptoms, especially with my memory lapses?"

Not only is it difficult to remember so many symptoms, it is also difficult to describe them. The women encounter shared obstacles to conveying the extreme character of their symptom composite. Many struggle to make their intense subjective distress intelligible and understandable to others. Their remarks are peppered with indications of these struggles.

Evelyn: Every time I try to do something it hurts. *It's hard to explain.*

Laura: *It is hard to describe.* It feels like my muscles are concrete that's beginning to set up or moving through concrete that's beginning to set up.

Robin: *It's really hard to explain* everything that goes along with it. When something goes around I catch it about three times. I really think it affects my immune system. I'm always sick, just *always* sick. My joints hurt and ache and I throw up all the time because of all the medicine. The quality of life I have right now is about zero.

Barbara: At least we know we are not dying from this. Although, I would have to say there are days when I thought I would rather die from this than have to live with it. It just gnaws at you sometimes; *it's hard to explain* how relentless it is.

One of the reasons it is so hard to explain FMS is because temporary episodes of the individual symptoms are recognized as mundane. Sufferers understand that it is the additive, intense, and persistent character of otherwise commonplace symptoms that distinguishes FMS and yet eludes cultural intelligibility. Recall Wendy's remarks that open this chapter. FMS is hard to explain "because there isn't any one thing you can put your finger on" but, rather, "it's everything in combination." Likewise, others report the difficulties they face when describing the non-routine character of their routine symptoms, or their abnormal reaction to what are generally recognized as normal complaints.

Jessica: My mother-in-law said to me, "So you have stress, pain, and fatigue. Everybody has stress, pain and fatigue." So you have to deal with that sort of thing all the time.

To deal with that sort of thing, many of the women with FMS specify the severity of their symptoms to differentiate them from run-of-the-mill complaints.

Margaret: I lose my thought in the middle of a sentence or I can't think of a common word, but more frequent than is "normal." It happens more than normal.

Doris: It is not just regular pain like everybody gets.

Sally: I know everyone gets tired but I'm talking about a different type of tired: drop dead tired.

In an effort to overcome the limitations of describing something so common and yet so extraordinary, the women assemble available metaphors and everyday images in an effort to speak in a framework of cultural intelligibility. Earlier, Laura described the sensation in her muscles as "concrete that's beginning to set up." The following are a few additional examples.

Evelyn: I feel like an old lady.

Robin: I feel like the tin man with no oil.

Courtney: There are days when you wake up feeling like you've worked a sixteen-hour day of manual labor.

Suzanne: I wake up and feel like I've been run over with a Mack truck, like somebody in the night just beat my body to a pulp.

Margaret: You feel like you have been run over by a Mack truck. Everybody uses that phrase because that is what it feels like. You can't move a muscle.

Multiple, commonplace complaints coalesce into a chronic and intense symptom composite that, at once, is acutely experienced and culturally elusive. As such, those who suffer grapple to translate comprehensibly for others that which is so obvious to them. Their efforts to do so capture the essence of what has been described as the paradox of pain. In her book *The Body in Pain: The Making and the Unmaking of the World*, Elaine Scarry (1985) describes how the intensity of pain as a subjective experience defies symbolic representation, thereby disallowing others to confirm its intensity or even its existence. The pain and related symptoms of FMS remain hard to explain because, as purely subjective realities, they resist symbolic transport from the private to the public world.

Functional Consequences: Daily Restrictions and Lives Interrupted

Describing the dramatic functional consequences of their FMS symptoms is a principal way sufferers concretize for others the force of their illness. Listening to women's descriptions of FMS is listening to a litany of daily restrictions and tales of lives interrupted. Women's lives change dramatically with FMS. Some highlight how even simple daily tasks, literally, become painstaking, whereas others reflect on the full range of loss that accompanies FMS.

Joyce: If I go to the store, I come home and I rest. I have a 600 square foot apartment but it takes me three days to clean. I dust one day and that is enough. I vacuum the next day and that is enough. That may be it for the day.

Robin: Just getting out of bed and getting a shower is a major accomplishment.

Courtney: Eventually you can no longer work. I am getting to the point now where I can hardly drive because of the pain and fatigue. It is very hard to deal with. You lose the quality of life because of the fibromyalgia.

Suzanne: Take your lifestyle, what you're doing right now and all of a sudden cut it in half. All of a sudden you cannot do even half of what you were able to do before. That changes your whole life.

Jessica: Fibromyalgia changes everything in your life. I can't do the things I use to do. I can't work. I can't travel. I can't take care of my family or even myself. Sometimes I can't even get out of bed. I can't, I can't, I can't! I could go on but you get the point.

Sufferers cut back on a growing number of daily activities, giving up dreams and chores alike, until eventually little or nothing is left to cut from their lives. Yet, despite their increasingly restrictive existence, their symptoms persist. What is more, with time, their symptoms and restrictions interact, resulting in a growing sense of hopelessness. As the distresses and limitations accrue in both number and severity, women find themselves caught in a downward spiral of disablement and despair. The following are typical recollections.

Betsy: It just got to the point where my whole body ached and I could not move. . . . I felt so bad that I wanted to die. I couldn't get off the couch. I didn't know what to do. I was at the end of my rope. I saw blackness all around me and I couldn't get out of it.

Valerie: My husband had to get me up in the morning and get me dressed. I was going from the bed to the chair. . . . The disease got to the point where I was eliminating everything out of my life. I stopped doing crafts, sewing, . . . anything that caused pain I stopped. Then one day I realized I was not doing anything. You find yourself in a tailspin and there's no end to it.

Both Betsy and Valerie, overwhelmed by the cumulative effect of symptoms, find themselves at the end of a frightening, unfolding story. Both women speak of falling out of their everyday world into utter nothingness. Physical and emotional torments are deeply interwoven as the sequence of events build to a crescendo: something has to give. Perhaps, for this reason, most of the women spoke of suicide, in either concrete or abstract terms; following are a few of many examples.

Phyllis: I got real bad and I was planning to die. To do something I guess. When the pain gets so bad I can't take it anymore. . . . I thought maybe I would run out in front of a car. Or thought I would drive into a semi head-on. It scares me. I would never do anything intentionally . . . but it gets so bad.

Alice: When I get real desperate, I sit here with all my pills together and think about trying to end it again. . . . Your mind won't shut off. Your body is hurting so bad.

Cindy: This [FMS] isn't going to kill me so that leaves only one way out, and you can't help but think that way from time to time.

In sum, women provide similar descriptions of FMS as a demoralizing set of functional restrictions. Their accounts blur disablement and despair as each begets the other. Further, their accounts reveal a common predicament of FMS: how to escape something that is experienced as fundamentally inescapable.

Symptom Variability: Baseline and Flare-ups

Women's descriptions of FMS also reliably include an account of its cyclical nature. Although FMS symptoms have a constant presence, from time to time the symptoms are exacerbated. For example, Suzanne explains the difference between the *baseline* and *flare-up* phases of FMS.

Suzanne: Fibromyalgia is this flulike feeling. If I could describe to you what it feels like, I would say it is like when you have the flu. You know when you have the flu and when your fever goes up and you feel all achy all over? You just hurt all over? Well, with fibromyalgia that's how I feel all the time; that's how I've felt all these years . . . and the feeling never goes away. That's called baseline pain and you get to a point that you can deal with that because it's just there all the time. The worst thing is that at different points in time you get flare-ups. Sometimes you can get sick and it can cause a flare-up; sometimes extra stress can cause a flare-up. Sometimes traumatic things, like car accidents, can cause a flare-up. So, through your course of things you have these flare-ups that come from time to time.

As with Suzanne, all the women in this study describe a dramatic difference in the intensity of their symptoms between the persistent baseline and periodic flare-ups or flares. The women move between these two states, lingering in one or the other for varying lengths of time. For example, some flares last several months, separated by longer periods of less pronounced dysfunction, as Ellen and Paula explain.

Ellen: I got real sick. I was sick from December until the end of March with flu and a sinus infection. Exactly four years later. . . the same thing happened again. I was sick for three months. I was so sick I had to crawl on my hands and knees up the steps and scoot down the stairs on my butt.

Paula: I usually have shorter episodes, you know, semifunctional six to nine months and then a period, maybe if I'm lucky, of eighteen months of pretty high functioning. Then flat on my back again.

In contrast to these longer flare states, symptom severity also fluctuates on a much shorter-term basis. Every few days, indeed day-to-day, symptoms and levels of functioning can change radically. Valerie and Alice provide characteristic descriptions of the more interim and routine ebb and flow in symptoms.

> **Valerie:** You're unable to function on a day-to-day basis. Some days you can't function at all, other days you function just fine.

> **Alice:** There are times when we feel better than other times. I can have three or four days when I can get up and function for blocks of time, maybe four hours at one time. Do something fun. There are other days when I can't get out of bed until ten or eleven and then I have to sit for a couple of hours and then I fall asleep for a couple of hours. And I'll have three or four days like that. I compare it to just existing on the bad days. I can't really call it living. I don't feel it's living; it's just existing trying to get through these days.

Movement between good and bad periods, good and bad days, is un-equivocally a part of the shared essence of the FMS illness experience. The following remarks further underscore this shared reality.

> **Hannah:** I just have good times and I have bad times. Like today, I'm feeling pretty good. I have other days that I feel like I can hardly drag myself through life, not to mention the pain.

> **Karen:** It's not always easy for my family to be understanding when I am having a bad day. Sometimes it is totally disabling. Other times it is something that you are able to live with.

> **Barbara:** There are good days and there are bad days. . . . There's always pain, maybe lower levels of it, but there's always pain. You kind of get used to it though. . . . On bad days it's unbearable. . . . On good days you still hurt but it's a lot different.

> **Doris:** There are some days where I feel great, where I am on top of everything and I think about getting a job, but other days you're just a vegetable. Some days, the bad days, where I'm in a lot of pain, it will take me hours to get dressed. A two o'clock appointment would be the earliest in the day that I could make an appointment. It's just crazy, and it's very hard to accept.

Whether a flare-up translates into a few bad months or a few bad days, it forces the individual either to slow down or shut down. As such, a flare undermines daily continuity and routine. In her book *Good Days/Bad Days*, Kathy Charmaz explores the ways living with the fluctuations of chronic illness shapes the experience of time. According to Charmaz (1991: 5), a "good day" permits a routine and "even schedule," whereas a "bad day" forces the individual to focus exclusively on the present and attend to "immediate needs." Courtney's description of her last flare provides a telling example of how a bad day with FMS undermines an agenda in favor of the here and now.

> **Courtney:** I would get out of bed and go have a shower, then I would go lie on the bed. Then I would dry myself and dry my hair, then I would rest again. Then I would get dressed, then I would rest again. Then I would come eat a bowl of cereal, and then rest again. It was awful.

Likewise, Phyllis vividly conveys the hopelessness that can result from being mired in the immediacy of overwhelming symptoms in contrast to the optimism of daily routine.

> **Phyllis:** I hurt all the time, but sometimes I hurt so badly I can't breathe.... You just never feel good. Never, never, never.... But sometimes, when I feel a little bit better, I feel like there is everything to live for. When I'm feeling bad I don't even really care if I live.

Although dealing with the immediacy of a flare turns routine activities into laborious struggles and dramatically slows the pace of daily life, the women in this study confront a more general consequence of their illness: the pace of their *entire* life must be slowed. Because overdoing it during periods of relative well-being can easily trigger a flare state, the "even schedule" permitted on good days must also be highly restricted.

> **Suzanne:** You have to learn to pace yourself. Even in those good times, you have to pace yourself and not overdo it or you can throw yourself into a flare-up.

> **Morgan:** I am doing a little better now than I was, but I want to keep it that way. That means living with limits because even little things can put me in a flare.

Consequently, whereas a flare corresponds to what Charmaz calls the "immersion in illness," or a total relinquishing of self and everyday life to the capriciousness of symptoms, restricting one's daily life during baseline periods to avoid future flare-ups becomes a *life founded on illness*. According to Charmaz (1991: 76), "[w]hen life becomes founded on illness, illness is not simply intrusive. No longer can people add illness to the structure of their lives; instead, they must *reconstruct* their lives upon illness."

Economy of the Body: Body Mindfulness, Self, and the Life World

As such, another core and shared feature of the FMS experience is developing the boundaries of a life founded on illness, which, simply stated, is a strategy for living within new restrictions and parameters concerning what type of life is possible. As the following comments reveal, sufferers understand that flare-ups are largely the result of transgressing these new restrictions and parameters.

> **Wendy:** There is just so much that I will never be able to do again. If you overdo and don't learn your own limitations with this disease, you will put yourself into a flare. You put yourself into a fog. You don't know whether you're coming or going and you are in so much pain. It is not worth it.

> **Margaret:** I have learned to recognize what is going on in my body. You need to know when you can't do things. I can tell if this is not a good day and then I say, "Okay, I am not going to do much today."

> **Joyce:** If I am not careful... if I am not paying attention and I don't listen to myself very well and I decide to do something, the flare-ups are acute.

Flare-ups, however, are complicated. Even as those who suffer seek to learn about and recognize their limitations, figuring out the nature and degree of transgression necessary to trigger a flare also involves figuring out a constantly changing set of equations. Evidence of this uncertainty is found in women's comments about the lack of predictability associated with their movement between baseline and flares.

> **Doris:** Fibromyalgia is a very cyclical illness. It's so cyclical because you can have good times and then really bad times and you can *never predict* when it's gonna strike.

> **Morgan:** I *can't predict* what I will feel like tomorrow, or next week, or even an hour from now. Flares come and go with no rhyme or reason. I figure out wine is a trigger and so I switch to Coke. Of course that doesn't work so I try something else.

> **Paula:** The problem with fibromyalgia is its total *lack of predictability*. There's only one thing you can predict... if you overdo it enough you will collapse. But you *can't predict* what enough is. One time you might get away with a whole lot and just pay for it a little. Another time you might get away with very little and pay and pay for it for months. You just don't know.

Although the course of FMS is not predictable; in fact, *because* the course of FMS is not predictable, women anxiously and determinedly attempt to develop a better framework for calculating their movement in and out of flare-ups. Interestingly, they do so using a common conceptual model in which the individual possesses a certain amount of physical "capital" that can be accumulated, spent, and overspent. Above, for example, Paula observes that "you might get away with a whole lot and pay only a little" or you might "get away with very little and pay and pay." Examining how sufferers construct this framework—a form of self-awareness that might aptly be called *the economy of the body*—is an illuminating way to see the impact of fibromyalgia on everyday life.

Within the framework of the economy of the body, time, activities, and suffering are all continually monitored and assessed, as captured in the following remarks.

> **Rachel:** On a good day, or good half day, you have weeks of stuff that had not been tended to and so you try to get as much done as you can. What you ask yourself is how much am I going to pay for this?

> **Mary:** Sometimes I just do things and then pay for it later.

> **Betsy:** I just take every day for what I can get out of it. I try to do that as much as I can, but I find that when I overdo it, I pay for it!

Activities are also traded off in a system of exchange in which doing certain activities requires saving up energy by foregoing current or future activities.

> **Alice:** I used to be busy every weekend and go out to the movie during the week. Now, maybe I get together with somebody for a few hours once a month. I have to rest up for two days to have a few hours of fun.

> **Evelyn:** If I go out and overdo it, I have to sleep for the whole next day.

> **Barbara:** I'll push myself and then a few days later I will fall apart and need a couple days of rest.

> **Joyce:** If I choose to do something . . . I choose to hurt. If I choose to hurt, then I have to plan ahead. If I go to a dance . . . I will have to rest for two days. The next few days I am flat on my back. You have to say, "Well, that was fun?" It is a choice.

Calculations and exchanges are made to "bank" energy for special occasions or important events and simply to manage day-to-day activities. The principle is to maintain a positive account balance, although there are activities whose costs exceed what can be saved in advance. Sometimes, those costs are assumed; other times, they are deferred.

> **Jessica:** I had my son's graduation and I wanted to be sure to be able to attend and I wanted to have his grandparents to the house for dinner after. I knew it was going to *cost* me but it was important. I rested for days before, but I still spent the week after graduation in bed.

> **Wendy:** I had to write a three-page letter today and my arms are killing me. I knew that that would be the only major thing I would be able to do today. So you pick and choose. You can only do one or two things a day and that is it for the day.

Paula: So you have to decide between a shower and fixing yourself something to eat. You need to decide between blow drying your hair and going to the grocery store, between keeping your nails trimmed and being able to open and sort through all the mail. Those people [with FMS] who have the most functionality you will find have also given up a whole lot of the activities that we as a society look at as fundamental. They *earn* their energy somewhere.

As seen in the earlier discussion regarding functional restrictions and lives interrupted, earning some energy by giving up fundamental activities is very much a part of the shared resonance of the FMS experience. For some sufferers, even simple daily tasks, such as showering and sorting mail, become too costly. But even for the most highly functioning, the ability to work full-time outside the home and assume primary responsibility for domestic tasks is unfeasible. Using the language of the economy of the body, the women speak about their efforts (often unsuccessful) to accommodate the demands of their work and domestic roles and obligations.

Courtney: I had tried to work, but there was just no way. One of the jobs I did after my diagnosis was to try to work three and a half hours every weekday afternoon, but all of the hours that I was not actually working I was lying on the couch. I couldn't do anything. I would come home and eat a bowl of cereal and lay on the couch. That lasted for about five weeks and I knew I just couldn't do it anymore. Anyway, so that's all there was to that.

Mary: I used to clean houses for people and that was very, very hard on me. It was awful hard, so I had to give that up. I just couldn't keep doing it; I would come home and I would be so miserable I would end up in bed for a couple of days, you know.

Sally: I am currently employed but I will never return to full-time work. I am back working again three days a week as a nurses' aid. I just worked the last three days in a row and now, after that, I am exhausted. I will spend the next several days in bed. I hurt so bad I could scream. But you have to survive. I can't do this for long.

Paula: Standing up and deciding that you are going to do your dishes until they were done could put you in the state of collapse for weeks. . . . I would clean house and then be down for six weeks. Then I'd need to clean house again [laughs]. I finally got that that was not a good pattern.

As described here, the economy of the body among those who suffer from FMS parallels Norma Ware's (1999) description of how chronic fatigue syndrome (CFS) sufferers understand the "payback" associated with overexertion. According to Ware, some who suffer from CFS live within their limits, whereas others knowingly take on activities with a high likelihood of leaving them to "pay the price." Ware explains how this strategy—cutting back on activities now or paying the price later— is incompatible with the demands of our overly rationalized society. In particular, the slowed or erratic functioning of patients with CFS is anti- thetical to a work world where attendance must be steady and tasks must be done at a predictable, if not also a rapid pace. Similar incompatibles are evident in the lives of those who suffer from FMS, as Joyce recounts.

> **Joyce:** I couldn't keep a job because I could not come into work when I was sick, and I was sick most of the time. I kept trying to keep a regular job. I started missing. Invariably, you are late because you can't get going. You miss a day here, you miss a day there, because you can't get out of bed. Businesses have everything structured. Weekends are with your partner and family, so you can't use them to catch up. It is hard to do it all. I went back to work, feeling pretty good, worked two days and, all of a sudden, I just could not do it. I could not take the noise. I could not take the people. I could not take anything. I cannot do this.

Ware (1999: 321–22) suggests that cutting back on activities in the workplace and in the home are "active efforts to counter, even undo, the effects of particular social influences on individual lives." More specifi- cally, Ware suggests that CFS is something of a strategic response to the burdens placed on women trapped between traditional ideals about wom- anhood and the demands of contemporary life. Ware's insights are valu- able in that they direct our attention to the existing tensions character- izing women's lives that can produce ill health. Nevertheless, there are limitations to the argument that CFS, and by extension FMS, is a practical way of negotiating the difficulties of "doing it all."

Whereas it is true that those who suffer from CFS or FMS curtail their obligations in response to their illness, they do so at tremendous costs to themselves. The economic and interpersonal losses are high. Careers and homes are lost; financial debts pile up; marriages, partnerships, and friendships become too strained to last; children feel neglected; and so- cial isolation can become a daily norm. Moreover, as women pull back from their work and domestic roles, there is a corresponding erosion of self-identity and self-worth. At best, women carve out something of a life for themselves despite FMS, not because of FMS. The comments of Laura and Valerie expose the difficulties of seeing FMS as an advantageous life strategy in the context of its resultant losses, including the mortification of self.[2]

> **Laura:** I couldn't work. I had to postpone getting married because I didn't want to be a burden to my fiancée. I sold so much stuff. I sold my big car and bought a little clunker. I even hocked stuff. That is stressful. . . . I have worked since I was sixteen years old. Your self-identity and your self-worth

and confidence . . . just fall. But you have to try and make some kind of life for yourself and that is so hard.

Valerie: Fibromyalgia affects how you feel about yourself. Your family sees this person that used to be able to do everything, who all of a sudden can't even prepare a meal. You have to work through all this emotional stuff. You have no self-esteem and yet you have to find a way to go on.

Whether FMS represents women's somatic resistance, conscious or unconscious, to the excessive and rationalized demands of society will not be resolved here. To be sure, the "economy of the body" is a metaphorical language that is widely encountered in the cultural landscape of capitalist society. It is a readily available and comprehensible way to speak about the restrictions that FMS implies and the corresponding meaning FMS symptoms have in women's everyday lives. Beyond this, however, the economy of the body provides a glimpse into something more all encompassing about the lived experience of FMS. Above all, it points to an acute *corporeal awareness* that is a fundamental and shared element of the FMS illness experience.

The woman who suffers must be fully conscious of her body and constantly calculate the bodily costs of activities. She must be continually attentive to her "account balance" by being fully aware of her body's status.

Morgan: I have to keep tabs on my energy by listening to my body all the time. It tells me what I can and can't do, but I got to listen. This disease has taught me to pay attention to my body and not push it. I heard someone talk about FMS being like a bowl of marbles. You have so many marbles and that's that. You can use a marble here, use a marble there, but you will lose all your marbles if you don't listen to your body [laughs]. That's fitting, because you really *do* lose your marbles if you don't watch out.[3]

Thus, the sufferer becomes aware of her body as an object, which she seeks to understand through ongoing dialogue. As case in point, sufferers like Joyce and Laura pay attention, listen, and talk to their bodies.

Joyce: My hips would be screaming at me so I just tell my hips, "Shhh, I hear you." I talk to my body a lot. I listen to it. At this point, we have a fifty-fifty deal. It is not going to run my life and I am not going to jeopardize it either.

Laura: I started paying attention and I realized that I did not straighten my legs. I started paying attention to how my body moved and I realized I did everything with my lower back muscles. Somewhere along the line all these muscles were guarded and not allowing other muscles to do what they were supposed to do. I had to start using imagery to think about what my body was doing.

This disposition toward *body mindfulness* makes sense given the immediacy of symptoms and the costs of inattention, namely a potential flare-up. At the same time, this disposition represents a marked break from what is taken for granted in everyday life. In effect, body mindfulness, expressed through the construct of the economy of the body, offers a way of coping with the numerous, intense, and unpredictable symptoms of FMS. At the same time, this benefit comes at a cost.

The Unmaking of the Life World

In the words of Peter Berger and Thomas Luckmann (1967: 22): "The reality of everyday life is organized around the 'here' of my body." We know the world is vast, but we experience our everyday lives primarily within a zone we can manipulate with our own bodies. Illness represents a break with the "until further notice" that characterizes the life world insofar as bodily symptoms separate us from those aspects of our everyday lives that ordinarily fall within our body's manipulative sphere. Indeed, the construction of social reality itself is impeded when symptoms significantly encumber our bodily movement and sever us from routine actions and practices. Sally describes FMS as just such an encumbrance: "I describe fibro as being detached from your external environment." Cindy succinctly notes, "My entire life is dealing with fibromyalgia symptoms."

The symptoms of FMS detach the sufferer from her routine practices. More and more time is focused on managing symptoms and less and less time on living in and through one's body at work, home, and play. In turn, the consequences of severe social restriction on self-identity are profound. Instead of the complex and elaborate social world in which the self becomes constituted via social actions, interactions, and performance, the world of those who suffer from FMS atrophies. Although the self is always an ongoing and contingent accomplishment (Berger and Luckmann 1967; Giddens 1991; Goffman 1959; Mead 1934), FMS sufferers lose access to many of the fields in which that accomplishment ordinarily transpires. In addition, available fields narrow significantly, further restricting the opportunities to engage in the ongoing work of self-construction. This is the most obvious way FMS represents the erosion of self and life world—one that is shared by sufferers of many other serious illnesses.

Not only do intense symptoms bar the sufferer from moving through her routine of daily life, they also force her into a state of consciousness in which she is always *with*—and yet always *against*—her body. The existence of this state of consciousness is another way in which FMS represents the demise of the taken-for-granted. Despite the body's determining role in moving us through our everyday lives, awareness of that reality ordinarily eludes us. Indeed, a characteristic part of the taken-for-granted life world is a fairly unmindful standpoint vis-à-vis the routine body. In contrast, when we are ill, we become aware of our routine body and, indeed, it can assume a constant presence in our consciousness. Drew Leder (1990) uses the phrase the "dys-appearing body" to capture our awareness of the body in illness in contrast to its disappearance in health. A lack of routine body awareness is the taken-for-granted privilege of health, whereas constant body mindfulness is a central cognitive template for those who suffer from FMS.[4]

Especially in conjunction with the inexact boundaries of FMS as a biomedical construct, there are important consequences of body mindfulness for shaping the FMS illness experience. Sufferers come to perceive and, in turn, know their bodies and actions progressively *through* the framework of FMS. Sleepless nights, dirty dishes, aches and pains, letter writing, changes in vision, marital discord, forgetfulness, drying one's hair—few sensations or daily activities fall fully outside the cognitive schema of FMS. This cognitive schema, therefore, is also a part of how FMS becomes a life founded on illness. Whatever else FMS may or may not be from a biomedical standpoint, it unquestionably operates as a cognitive structure through which much of life is organized, managed, experienced, and given meaning.

Conclusion

Although no shared, objective biomedical indicator exists for FMS, it is described in very similar ways as a subjective illness experience. For example, although it is hard for sufferers to explain, FMS symptoms are experienced as overwhelming as a result of their collective breadth and intensity. The subsequent disablement and despair are likewise part and parcel of the FMS experience. Moreover, whereas there is a constant presence of baseline symptoms, sufferers describe a dramatic and unpredictable amplification of those symptoms during periods called flare-ups. Managing both the baseline and flare-up symptoms of FMS requires that women significantly restrict their activities, including reducing or withdrawing from their work and domestic obligations, which results in a predictable erosion of self-worth. Finally, these restrictions are constantly assessed, reassessed, and managed through the development of corporeal mindfulness. In sum, the symptomatic features of FMS represent a rupture in what is taken-for-granted in everyday life and leave in its stead a cognitive schema that incessantly organizes bodily perceptions within its parameters.

Independent of the biomedical reality of FMS, the idea of FMS thus stretches out to bracket, bind, and bestow meaning to a vast array of experiences and to mold routine behaviors. This process reifies FMS itself; that is, it makes FMS appear to be something other than, or more than, a conceptual category around which experience is organized. This is central to the social reality of FMS.

5

In Search of Meaning

or those who suffer from fibromyalgia syndrome (FMS), the world is divided into those who accept FMS as "real" and those who do not; the former are friends, the latter are foes.[1] The division of the world into these two opposing factions grows out of a set of encounters that characterizes the FMS experience. Every woman's FMS story includes a struggle to have her symptoms recognized as real in the face of disbelief. In particular, a central thread running through women's FMS narratives is the weaving together of illness onset and a fruitless search for its medical meaning. Their symptoms appear; they seek medical counsel; and doctors are unable to find anything wrong or offer palliative treatment. Moreover, this thwarted enterprise is usually protracted. Most patients with fibromyalgia experience five to seven years of symptoms before a diagnosis is made (Goldenberg 1999). In this respect, the women in this study are typical. They endured an average of six and a half years of acute symptoms prior to diagnosis.

This chapter examines the central importance of the prolonged and frustrating search for symptom meaning to the FMS experience. In brief, women sufferers are caught between their symptoms and science: they experience their symptoms as unmistakably real, whereas physicians find "nothing wrong." Moreover, the coming together of women's symptomatic certainty and biomedical doubt is constantly mediated by a gender ideology that presupposes women's irrationality and emotional volatility, which powerfully shapes what is said and heard within the clinical context. Women sufferers feel both bewildered and discredited as a result of these interactions. In this way, FMS represents a threat to the sufferer's taken-for-granted assumptions about her body and reality, and their relationship to one another.

Meaning Quest: Life World Versus the World of Biomedicine

A universal feature of the illness experience is the search for symptom meaning. At nearly the same moment we become aware of our symptoms, we become interested in knowing what they signify. When we wake up in the morning with a headache and congestion, we consider the possibility that we are coming down with a cold or flu and, as the day proceeds, we either confirm or reject our earlier assessment on the basis of the unfolding status of our symptoms. If illness is symptomatically confirmed, we may make changes in our behavior or administer remedies. We are also likely to construct an explanation for why we have become ill: we are run down, came into close contact with someone who has a contagious illness, and the like. Puzzling about what our symptoms mean and responding to them therapeutically bring into play local orientations and knowledge. Because of biomedicine's cultural dominance, this includes basic biomedical information that effectively circulates as taken-for-granted. For example, being run down and being exposed to infection draw on commonsense applications of immunological and bacteriological or virological knowledge, respectively. Insofar as our illness is routine, trivial, and temporary, these local frameworks, inflected with lay interpretations of biomedicine, are adequate for making sense of our experience.

In contrast, if our illness is not mundane and fleeting, we recognize that we alone do not possess the necessary knowledge to understand or respond to our symptoms. Instead, we culturally recognize this matter as falling legitimately within the jurisdiction of biomedicine. We assume physicians will translate our symptom experience into medical knowledge by offering us a diagnosis and treatment. In the case of FMS, however, such a translation is typically not forthcoming, leaving the sufferer in an epistemological and emotional tailspin in which the disruption of daily life that commonly accompanies any serious illness intensifies into a full-blown crisis of confidence.

A common difficulty those with FMS confront is the disparity between the natural attitude of everyday life and the scientific attitude of biomedicine. Whereas everyday knowledge, based on the certainty of subjective experience, suspends doubt, biomedical knowledge, based on objective evidence, suspends belief. The medical encounter brings together these two disparate perspectives, or what Elliot Mishler (1984: 14) calls "voices." Patients bring the "voice of the life world," which represents the taken-for-granted assumptions about reality, whereas physicians bring the "voice of medicine," which represents a host of technical and scientific suppositions concerning reality. These distinct voices are based on different assumptions and are granted unequal levels of authority within the medical encounter. For the individual sufferer, the very perception of embodied distress confirms its existence (beyond doubt); in the clinical context, however, the life-world voice is subordinate and awaits translation into the authoritative voice of medicine.

The suppositions through which biomedicine translates subjective reality into biomedical reality are dependent on the observable and measurable body. In particular, disturbances that can be seen in the body (either directly or indirectly via scientific instrumentation) are *real* illnesses. Conversely, illnesses that cannot be so observed are suspected of existing only in the minds of those who suffer; that is, they are suspected of being *not real.* This set of assumptions is premised on the conceptual division between the body and mind and can be traced to the seventeenth century philosopher René Descartes. Because all physical things can be measured in terms of the physical space they occupy, Descartes reasoned that the mind could not be a physical thing. After all, the mind (i.e., thoughts, feelings, and desires) does not exist spatially. Thus, Descartes deduced that the physical and mental worlds of the individual were distinct, an idea we now call the Cartesian mind-body dualism. This division became increasingly significant as biomedicine began to place more and more emphasis on the observable body. In fact, adherence to the mind-body dualism, in conjunction with increasingly sophisticated ways of observing the body, is a central mechanism by which biomedicine gained cultural authority during the nineteenth and twentieth centuries and it continues to account for biomedicine's contemporary power, prestige, and legitimacy.

Both Paul Starr (1982) and Michel Foucault (1975) place an emphasis on the accumulation of corporeal data through scientific instrumentation as a key factor in the history of medicine's cultural ascendancy. With the invention of the stethoscope by René Laennec in 1819, for example, physicians gained empirical information about their patients that patients themselves could not provide. Scientific instrumentation allowed what Foucault called the "medical gaze" to move beyond the surface of the body and a patient's subjective description of his or her symptoms to gather objective measurements of diseases that lie "in the secret depths of the body" (Foucault 1975: 136). As physicians expanded or deepened their gaze, they also expanded the information asymmetry between themselves and patients and, in turn, increased their power and authority

(Starr 1982). At the same time that patients became dependent on physicians to interpret their bodies via instrumentation, physicians freed themselves from a reliance on patients' interpretative accounts of sickness and distress. Physicians' facts, not patients' sensations, served as the principal basis for determining bodily reality. Of course, the stethoscope was merely an early step in a rapid process that remains both ongoing and astonishing.

Biomedical Unmaking of the Life World

The mind-body dualism and the corresponding detachment of biomedical knowledge from a patient's subjective report via the ever-penetrating gaze frame the FMS experience. Indeed, these core features of biomedicine account for the similarity in tone and sequence of medical encounters described by women sufferers. First, sufferers confirm that an illness or injury is somewhat serious or persistent and make an appointment to see their general practitioner. Their general practitioner, however, finds nothing remarkable in routine diagnostic work-ups and so initiates a chain of referrals. By and large, the women move from specialist to specialist on a more or less symptom-by-symptom basis: gastroenterologists for stomach distress; neurologists for migraines and cognitive dysfunction; gynecologists for menstrual symptoms and vaginal or bladder infections; and rheumatologists for musculoskeletal pain. Along the way, some women find modest or temporary remedies for discrete complaints. Nevertheless, despite the growing number of specialists engaged, no explanations are found for their systemic illness and their general health does not improve.

> **Wendy:** I had MRIs [magnetic resonance imaging], bone scans, epidurals, nerve blocks. I had done everything. I went to two pain clinics. Shrinks. Probably everyone you've interviewed with fibromyalgia will tell you the same thing. You have to go from doctor to doctor to doctor. It was one nightmare after another, one doctor after another.

Indeed, nearly all the women said the same thing.

> **Robin:** I've been to about every kind of doctor there is, and I'm not kidding.

> **Courtney:** I had tests from every kind of a doctor you can imagine. They sent me to osteopaths, to the psychiatrist, everything. Every kind of a doctor you could name I went to see.

> **Laura:** I have gone from doctor to doctor trying to find out what was wrong with me.

Paula: I've seen neurologists, osteopaths, oral surgeons. I can't think of all the different kinds of medicine that there are, but I have seen pretty much the gamut of referrals. Gastroenterologists, gynecologists, if it's got an "ologist" behind it I've probably seen them.

Emily: I started with my primary care physician. . . . After that I went to every doctor known to man.

Negative test results, puzzled doctors, mistaken diagnoses, and ineffective remedies accumulate in a frustrating sequence. Mary, for example, describes searching for an answer and treatment for the severe pain and weakness in her hands that forced her to quit her job as a cashier.

Mary: My doctor tested for all kinds of things. He tried a cortisone shot for my pain, but that did nothing. Since he couldn't find anything wrong, he sent me to a neurologist. They thought that at first it might be carpal tunnel. It wasn't carpal tunnel. Then they thought maybe it was a [pinched] nerve. I went to one doctor after another. I also went to an orthopedic doctor. None of it worked. . . . I went through six weeks of physical therapy. They tried all sorts of electrical gadgets. At the end of the six weeks they put my hands in hot wax. That didn't work. I tried another four weeks of therapy. It didn't work either.

Margaret similarly describes a ten-year period where she bounced between baffled doctors and ineffective medications.

Margaret: I had been going to rheumatologists and I had shifted from one to the other. Each would tell me, "I can't do anything for you, go see somebody else." I had been doing this for years and getting what I call the "wonder drug of the month." That one didn't work; that one made you sleep all day; that one made you throw up. Every month I would go back to some doctor and get some new drug.

In sum, the women describe a cycle of doctors, tests, treatments, and uncertainties that, with only minor variation, repeat themselves over and again. This cycle is captured succulently, and with good humor, by Sally in a portrayal of her fourteen-year trek from doctor-to-doctor in search of an explanation for her disabling constellation of symptoms: "Round and round she goes and where she stops no one knows."

"Nothing Is Wrong"

In the process of these ineffectual medical encounters, the evidence builds: there is *no* evidence for their illness. The disparity between overwhelming symptoms and a procession of negative test results is bewildering. Over time, the fissure between the certainty of one's symptoms and the lack of proof of their existence creates more and more discord.

Jessica: I had x-rays of my entire body, CAT [computed axial tomography] scans, bone scans, ultrasounds, blood test after blood test after blood test. I had upper and lower GIS [gastrointestinal]. I have had a few MRIs. There isn't a part of my body that some doctor or another did not test trying to find out what was wrong. Nothing, nothing was wrong! Nothing, except I couldn't get out of bed!

Doris: I had two MRIs. . . . Then I had x-rays and blood work. It was always pretty good. It shows that you're in good health. But at the same time you're running into things and stumbling and losing your short-term memory.

Betsy: The doctors did all kinds of tests on me to try to figure out what it was, but nothing would show up. It was so frustrating to me, because I felt sick, I felt ill, and they just basically kept saying that there was nothing wrong with me.

With good reason, patients become angry and anxious over this inconsistency. How can their symptoms be nothing? There simply has to be an answer! Nevertheless, answers elude both the doctors and sufferers.

Rachel: After I was in the [psychiatric] hospital for nineteen days, after they let me out of the nut ward, I was so angry. What is this? This is *something!*

Cindy: I was getting angry because the doctors would all be looking at me and tell me there was nothing wrong. I would go home crying every time and ask myself "what the [hell] is this?"

Evelyn: I was angry. They make you think there's *nothing* wrong with you!

In one case after another, the women are left to reconcile the discrepancy between symptoms that are unmistakably real to them and an expanding medical record that finds *nothing wrong*. In general, the women switch between two equally anxious states: one in which they fear their doctors failed to detect something terrible, and the other in which they question their own sanity. With respect to the former, Jessica and Alice's experiences are illustrative.

Jessica: I would go to bed at night and fear I was dying of bone cancer. I would become so convinced that I could feel it crawling up my spine. Well, why did I have so much pain? Maybe my doctor missed it.

Alice: I would go through medical books page by page, trying to see if anything would fit. The closest thing I could come up with was a brain tumor. Nearly everyone in my [immediate] family and extended family has had cancer. I figured I was dying of cancer.

With respect to the latter, at some point the women begin to doubt their own sanity. Indeed, it is difficult not to. Many women report internal conversations that give voice to their own suspicions and misgivings. The following statements are typical in this regard.

Hannah: Because I was feeling pain down my legs, they sent me to a neurologist. I had a whole work-up by a neurosurgeon and had an MRI. He also did blood work and, of course, he couldn't find anything wrong with me. So, it was about that time that I started thinking, "Well, what is wrong with me?"

Suzanne: You feel like you're crazy, losing your mind. I have been through a lot. Nobody would ever want to have this. Not all this pain and fatigue. You start to think, "Well, maybe I'm just going crazy. Is it all in my head or not?"

Doris: I was convinced that I must have been crazy. How could I hurt so bad and the doctors not know what it was from?

Women's apprehensions about their hold on reality intensify with each medical interaction that ends with the proclamation "there is nothing wrong." Even while physicians use this phrase to capture their technical inability to find any organic dysfunction, it is clearly embedded with implicit mind-body assumptions. Physicians often use this phrase, and patients usually hear it, as an accusation that the symptoms in question are not real, but rather an imaginary byproduct of mental instability. Both parties in the doctor-patient dyad quickly understand the implications of multiple clinical visits and the absence of any visible organic dysfunction. Invariably, practitioners up and down the referral chain begin to assume that women's symptoms are psychogenic. So begins a new string of referrals to mental health providers and prescriptions for psychotropic medications. In the process women feel invalidated.

Maude: I have been going to doctors since I was eighteen and I am forty-nine now. They would try to help but then they would give up. They have just been passing me on, giving me more and more antidepressants.

Paula: I didn't see [any] doctors for nine years. They weren't helping me. They kept sending me to psychiatrists. Damned if I was going to go back!

As a matter of course, the women describe a succession of interactions in which they feel doctors dismiss their physical complaints as mental, emotional, or personal problems. The following comments capture these common grievances.

Robin: There was a woman doctor I went to and she would give me a paper bag, make me sit in the hall, and breathe in that [the bag] while she would massage my shoulders. That was her idea of helping me. I would say, "Look, you know I can't even turn my head."

Suzanne: The rheumatologist was convinced that I was going through marriage problems. But there were no problems at the time; everything was going really well. We'd never had any marriage problems. But the rheumatologist was convinced, because he didn't know what was wrong. So, "it has to be stress, or it must be your marriage, so maybe you need to see a psychotherapist." That's fine and I'm not against seeing them, but it was very obvious to me that he was not listening to me. When I told him that we did not have any marriage problems, he just didn't want to hear that because that would be saying that he didn't know what was wrong with me.

Courtney: You are already so down that you can barely get from one day to the next and then you have a doctor telling you you're crazy! Then, they make you pay for that! A lot of them nod and pat you on the head, but then ignore what you are saying.

Sufferers feel that physicians fail to listen to them or take them seriously and, as a result, they are left to endure their disabling symptoms, personal humiliation, and challenges to their subjective experience of reality. The union of symptoms and medical disparagement represent what Leslie Cooper (1997) calls a "double disruption" to everyday life. As with sufferers of other illnesses that cannot be confirmed biomedically, the women bear the weight of their symptoms in want of cultural meaning and legitimacy. Suzanne and Courtney articulate the burdens of this double disruption as they expand on their above comments.

Suzanne: Enough already. You're dealing with this pain you have all the time. I do not have a day without pain. Dealing with that and *then* having somebody tell me I'm mental because they don't understand.

Courtney: You feel so defeated. . . . You are already so exhausted and so ill, and in so much pain, and here are these people hammering into your head, "There's nothing wrong with you. Go home, find an interest, get a hobby."

Courtney's comments, in particular, hint at what many FMS sufferers believe to be true—namely, that the failure on the part of physicians to listen to them or take them seriously is largely the result of cultural beliefs that interpret women's complaints as fanciful and equate women with irrationality. In the absence of clear biological signs for symptom distress, this ideology hangs over the medical encounter. Most of the women tell of situations where their complaints are trivialized and they are personally written off as overly emotional, neurotic, or hysterical.

Hannah: A rheumatologist kinda brushed me off because when I went into him I was pretty miserable. When he walked into the office, I burst into

tears, so he thought I was just nuts. He told me, "Oh, you just need to go
to your doctor and get an antidepressant." Anyway, he just brushed me off.
I guess he thought I was just another neurotic lady. So, I didn't go back to
him because he wasn't very sympathetic to my needs.

Morgan: From 1990 to 1998 I saw lots of doctors and a lot of them treat you
like you're just some unhappy housewife. I mean, I stopped telling doctors
that I felt depressed and I did my best not to cry in front of them because
I wanted them to listen to me.

Emily: A gastroenterologist said that it was just "female problems." That's
what he said!

Jessica: They tell you that you have "female problems." I had a lot of doctors
tell me that. So you go from doctor to doctor because you are not going
to go to one that tells you this kind of stuff. It just makes you furious.
You complain about back pain, and they do a pregnancy test. If that is
negative, they give you Prozac. They make you feel crazy! One doctor told
me I should try to get pregnant again, like what I needed was a happy
distraction or something. It just makes you furious.

Women become angry when their complaints are simultaneously feminized and psychologized. What is more, they respond by searching for
a more sympathetic doctor. As a rule, they abandon practitioners who
frame their disabling symptoms as psychosomatic or treat them as hysterical women. Laura, for example, never returned to her family physician
after his cavalier response to her pain that was so severe she was unable
to walk.

Laura: My family physician found two degenerating disks in my neck and
some degenerative changes in the middle of my back. He said, "Well, you
are getting into your late forties; you've got some degenerative changes
that come with age, so learn to live with it." He also gave me a prescription
for Paxil without giving me any of the tests for anxiety. I did not particularly
like his approach so I went to another doctor.

Others similarly tell of dropping doctors that dismiss their complaints
as psychological and moving on in search of one who is more willing to
listen.

Morgan: For eight years I went from doctor to doctor and they're all alike.
They are nice at first but before too long they come to the conclusion
you're a few bricks shy and when that happens you move on because it is
clear they're not listening to you any more.

Doctors' implicit or explicit suggestions that symptoms are psychogenic is, by far, the most common way women feel dismissed in the
clinical context. Many also feel invalidated when physicians frame their

predicament as a weight problem or the result of an inadequate level of physical fitness.

Phyllis: Medical doctors want to blame everything on depression. If they don't wanna blame it on depression, they wanna blame it on your weight.

Ellen: I kept going to doctors and they kept saying, "You're fat, lose weight, exercise. You'll be fine. Lose weight, exercise, you'll be fine." Do you know how many doctors told me that? I want to slap them!

Cindy: The rheumy [rheumatologist] started telling me how much better I'd feel if I went to aerobics class or something and got some weight off, that it would help my hip [pain]. Geez, I couldn't even move and he thinks I should do jazzercise!

Joyce: I have heard it so much. The doctors say, "You would feel better and have more energy if you just lost some weight." Okay, fine. I have been on about every program. I would lose sixty, seventy, eighty pounds, down to a weight I could not maintain. Well, I looked good, but I still hurt and I was still tired.

Overall, an unpromising sequence of medical encounters leaves women feeling ignored, demeaned, and discredited, as their deeply felt symptoms are framed as psychogenic, an over-reaction to personal or emotion problems, or the outcome of weight gain and physical inactivity. When patients feel discredited in these ways, the particular doctor-patient relationship is no longer sustainable. FMS sufferers are overwhelmingly women; their doctors—especially rheumatologists and other specialists to whom they are referred—are primarily men (American Medical Association 2004).[2] As such, their invalidation is structurally gendered, despite the individual personalities and beliefs of the particular players. In other words, a woman need not be hysterical and a doctor need not be sexist for the drama to unfold as though one or both were true. Both the social structure and context of the interaction are often of equal or greater significance in the exchange than the particulars of the individuals occupying the roles in the social plot.

The Other Side of the Doctor-Patient Relationship

It is important to recognize that these remarks come from only one of the two parties in the doctor-patient dyad. It is impossible to know how accurately these women have described their medical encounters, or if the encounters they have described are typical of those experienced by other FMS sufferers. Indeed, only by studying medical encounters directly can researchers comment with any degree of certainty about the character of doctor-patient interactions. Nevertheless, we can situate women's comments in studies about physician attitudes toward patients with med-ically unexplainable symptoms and conditions that fail to respond to standard treatment regimens.

Physicians are trained to value objective disease over and above sub-jective illnesses, and these values are part and parcel of the institutional world in which they establish their professional identities. As noted, lim-ited professional prestige is associated with treating patients with unspec-ified alignments or caring for those whose symptoms fail to improve with established medical protocols. In general, physicians evaluate such pa-tients as problematic, in large measure because they represent a barrier to their enactment of the ideal medical professional (i.e., one who ther-apeutically solves patients' objective medical problems). In some very basic ways, therefore, dealing with patients with medically uncertain ill-nesses represents a threat to professional identity (Asbring and Narvanen 2003). Moreover, physicians make moral judgments about patients with unexplainable symptoms (Freidson 1971), judgments that are height-ened in their interactions with women patients. For example, doctors routinely evaluate women's symptoms as more psychosomatically derived than men's and are more likely to suggest that women exaggerate symp-toms (Hoffmann and Tarzian 2001; Wallen et al. 1979).

We can also situate women's comments in existing research about in-teractions between doctors and women patients. For example, Howard Waitzkin (1991) finds that social problems that concern women are some-times raised in clinical encounters, by either patients or physicians, but the character of the encounter constrains physicians' responses and ac-tions. Physicians may not be oblivious to the ways social problems can adversely impact women's well-being, but they do not have a therapeutic remedy for women's low wages, patriarchal marriages, or the demands and drudgery of domestic labor. Most, however, do have a genuine de-sire to aid their troubled patients and, so, explains Waitzkin (1991: 141), they do what they can: "A tranquilizer provides a technical means of coping with a variety of bodily and emotional discomforts." We can see how Waitzkin's description of physicians' constrained efforts could leave women sufferers feeling discredited.

Thus, although one-sided, the descriptions of medical encounters pro-vided by women sufferers are not inconsistent with what is known about the character of medical work, the threat to professional identity that patients with unexplainable and untreatable symptoms represent, the moralism physicians exhibit toward such patients, and interactional dy-namics between doctors and women patients. What is more, whether women's impressions about the invalidating outcome of their medical encounters are fully accurate is less important to the FMS story than the fact that, in large numbers, women walk away from similar medical encounters feeling invalidated.

At first glance, the way women describe feeling dismissed by doctors "as women" might seem to contradict the central claim of Chapter 2, namely that biomedicine has not paid sufficient attention to issues of gender when it comes to FMS. From these descriptions, it appears as if physicians are willing to complicate the clinical encounter by raising social and personal issues of a gendered nature that may have an impact on women's well-being, even as women patients read this as dismissive of their "real" problems. But while this chapter speaks to micro-level doctor–patient interactions, Chapter 2 is concerned with the conceptual creation of FMS as a category of biomedical knowledge. In effect, these two chapters highlight the difference between clinical practice (emphasized in this chapter) and clinical research (emphasized in Chapter 2). Although both domains are guided by shared assumptions, clinical research is even more disconnected from the social contexts of its subjects than is clinical practice. The strict demands of research design preclude addressing exogenous complexities far more than do individual doctor-patient encounters.

Nevertheless, it is interesting to note that this difference is of little practical consequence, given the constraints of the clinical encounter portrayed above. Again, referring to the work of Waitzkin, although gender issues may get raised in interactions between doctors and women patients, gender issues are seldom, if ever, meaningfully addressed. To a large extent, therefore, the outcome of the clinical encounter between women patients and their doctors obscures the link between gender and women's health no less than the protocols of clinical research. Thus, these details do not fundamentally contradict the earlier claim that biomedicine has paid insufficient attention to issues of gender when it comes to FMS.

The Body and the Social Construction of Reality

When doctors are unable to translate women's subjective symptoms into objective biomedical evidence, a requisite foundation of everyday reality is threatened. From a sociological perspective, Peter Berger and Thomas Luckmann (1967: 1) explain, "real" phenomena are those things "we recognize as having a being independent of our own volition." When it comes to things that are "real," in other words, we are unable to simply "wish them away." Commonsense knowledge assures us our bodies are real. We can hardly doubt the existence of our arms and legs, given that we directly perceive, manipulate, and sense them. When it comes to our arms and legs, in short, we cannot simply wish them away. Accordingly, the body functions as a basis for the construction of everyday reality itself. The experience of our body, although perhaps not fully conscious to us in the state of health, is quintessentially valid. It exists beyond our volition. Even though we cannot see our back pain, we know it, through sensation, to be fundamentally real. At the level of experience then, the impartiality and immediacy of our body assures its reality. We accept our body's sensations as unconditionally real, suspending any doubt to the contrary. Again, that is, until further notice.

When women's corporeal certainty cannot be confirmed in biomedical terms, they discover they no longer feel confident about what is real and what is not. After all, if they cannot be certain that their own bodily sensations are real, about what can they be certain? Cindy, who injured her back working as a certified nurse assistant, shares her emotions after enduring more than three years of constant pain, dizziness, and headaches for which doctors had no explanation.

> **Cindy:** You are so confused and upset because nothing adds up or makes sense. I would cry and cry, just sit and cry because if all of this isn't real.... It's really scary.

What is scary is that as the sureness of the body is called into question, so too is reality itself. What is *real*? How is one to *know*? Although these questions are of perennial interest to philosophers, most people do not ordinarily raise them as they go about their everyday lives. Again Berger and Luckmann explain (1967: 2): "The man on the street does not ordinarily trouble himself about what is 'real' to him and about what he 'knows.'...He takes his 'reality' and his 'knowledge' for granted." This is the normal state of affairs "unless he is stopped short by some sort of problem."

Undeniably, women sufferers are stopped short by some sort of problem. They begin to wonder if they actually inhabit and experience the same world everyone else inhabits and experiences. These sufferers, once again, replay an intense internal dialogue, asking themselves questions about which there should be no doubt—their experiential sense of reality. Barbara and Emily's self-questioning is characteristic.

> **Barbara:** What is wrong with me? Why are all these things happening to me? Does everyone else feel like this and I'm just a wimp? I can't even begin to explain the stuff that you go through.

> **Emily:** I mean after you hear it enough you begin to question it. Is it in my head? Do I really feel this? Because I heard that from several doctors, "Its just growing pains, you'll grow out of it. Everyone deals with this kind of thing." So I started to think, well, maybe I just don't know how to deal with pain if everyone else can.

Jessica poses a similar question to herself nearly a year after the death of her five-year-old son, which resulted in the intensification of her long-standing pain and fatigue.

> **Jessica:** Then you start to wonder, "Is this all in my head?" Once you hear that over and over again, you can't help but wonder. "You're just upset about your son. You will get over it in time." So you start to wonder yourself. Well, maybe I am just upset about my son. Well, of course I am upset about my son! Maybe everyone else just handles things better than I do.

Barbara, Emily, and Jessica labor with truly unsettling and frightening thoughts. Maybe they are not like everyone else. Maybe they do not experience the world like everyone else. These distressing ideas lay bare the intersubjective basis of everyday reality. We assume that we share our everyday world with others, that there is a commonsense, natural attitude that we collectively hold. Berger and Luckman (1967: 23) explicate this attitude:

> I am alone in the world of my dreams, but I know that the world of everyday life is as real to others as it is to myself. . . . I know that my natural attitude to the world corresponds to the natural attitude of others. . . . The natural attitude is the attitude of commonsense consciousness precisely because it refers to a world that is common to many.

But what happens if an individual finds him- or herself doubting the extent to which he or she shares the natural attitude of others? Given that the suspension of such doubt is precisely what constructs what is taken for granted of everyday life, raising misgivings can result in its deconstruction. This is the state of affairs for women sufferers who find themselves unsure about their placement in what they had assumed to be a shared social reality. They feel more and more alien in a world they thought they understood and believed was consensual. Yet, precisely because their social reality is under siege, the women resolutely defend against its ruin.

The Reconstruction of Social Reality

Key to women's strategy for reclaiming their location in the consensual world is discounting previous psychogenic interpretations of their illness. Successfully completing this task begins to resolve difficult questions concerning their mental credibility and their grip on reality. For instance, because most of the women had psychiatric evaluations as part of the sequence of medical referrals, they evoke these appraisals as proof of their mental stability.

Jessica: They could not find anything wrong with me so they keep sending me back to shrinks but the shrinks would just tell me that I was sad about Jason [her recently deceased son]. I was just sad, not crazy. I have seen many, many psychiatrists and they say, "Well, you're not crazy."

Suzanne: My general practitioner didn't think it was a psychological problem so . . . I did not go to a psychiatrist at that time. He [her general practitioner] did an evaluation of his own . . . and he really didn't feel like there were any psychological problems.

Valerie: The doctors would say, "You have had a lot of stress. You should see a psychologist." I went to see a psychologist and it was helpful but the psychologist's diagnosis was that this was not a mental thing. Mentally, I am very stable. I have got good coping mechanisms.

The women also continue to reject the feasibility of a psychogenic explanation through their own analyses of their personal battles with depression and anxiety. Nearly all of the women in this study are depressed and most are anxious; many are diagnosed as such, whereas others merely acknowledge these as common states they experience to greater or lesser degrees. Nevertheless, there is a logical coherence in denying that their symptoms are psychosomatic, despite their high rates of psychological distress. Depression and anxiety, they conclude, are merely normal reactions to their relentless symptoms and the strain associated with managing medical uncertainty. These three comments are some of the many that capture the prevalent view among sufferers that mental distress is not the cause but the effect of the illness.

Suzanne: If I was depressed at all, it was at not knowing what was wrong with me, but it wasn't a *real* depression.

Laura: You show me someone who has been through what I have been through, and I will show you someone that is anxious.

Sally: Going in to the doctors and having them all tell you there is nothing wrong with you . . . it is no wonder we have high rates of psychiatric illness. I was never on psychiatric meds before fibro. The pain load, day after day, month after month, year after year, and it has been five years for me now. It is a full time job managing the pain. If the rates of psychiatric illness are high among those with FMS, it makes sense. I did not get fibro because I was nuts; I got nuts because of fibro.

Women's interpretation of their mental health problems as a secondary response also allows them to deflect another potentially discrediting detail. Nearly every woman in this study takes antidepressants as a part of her treatment protocol. Indeed, antidepressants are virtually the only treatment option to demonstrate clinical efficacy among patients with FMS, creating a situation in which the response to treatment itself can serve as proof of mental illness. The women resolve this contradiction not only by highlighting the wear and tear of enduring symptoms and medical disbelief, but also by specifying that a low dosage of antidepressants is often used to regulate sleep in patients with FMS, not to treat depression *per se*.

Mary: I am on a very low dose; they say it helps you get into a deeper sleep.

Barbara: My doctor prescribed an antidepressant. In low doses they help you to sleep.

It makes sense that women would be particularly sensitive to this issue, given that taking antidepressants potentially bolsters the claim that their illness is mental rather than physical in nature. Moreover, most of the women feel antagonistic toward doctors who, over the years, have sent them home with little but the newest mood-altering drug in response to their lengthy reports of debilitating symptoms. Such antagonism is likely warranted.

These women's individual experiences are borne out in research that demonstrates a well-established tendency on the part of physicians to see women's pain complaints as psychogenic and men's as organic and, correspondingly, their propensity to treat the former with antidepressants and anti-anxiety medications and treat the latter with painkilling narcotics. Clinically speaking, women's pain is treated less aggressively than men's, even when it has a known organic cause (e.g., cancer or surgical pain) (Hoffmann and Tarzian 2001). Women are more likely to be given anti-anxiety medications after coronary artery bypass surgery than pain-killing narcotics for postoperative pain and discomfort (Calderone 1990). Physicians' tendencies to treat women's pain as psychosomatic, even when obvious organic causes are at play, are considerably amplified when no clear explanations are found for the pain.

As a consequences of these circumstances, several women in this study face an ongoing struggle to get the medications necessary to keep their pain in check, whereas not one women feels similarly blocked from antidepressant or anti-anxiety medications. Valerie summarizes the general problem.

Valerie: It has been a long battle. My primary physician will not give me the pain medication I have asked for. I have a deteriorated disk in my neck and so finally he said he would give me a few pills for that. I went back to him and told him that because of this one little pill that I take a couple of times a day I am able to get my life back. If I don't take that medicine I cannot function. Managing the pain is the most important thing and physicians don't see that. They will give you antidepressants ... and they try to manage your other symptoms but they don't take care of the real problem, which is pain.

Sufferers also discount psychogenic interpretations of their condition by stressing the gender bias that characterizes their failed medical encounters. Physicians' failure to provide a specific biomedical explanation for women's symptoms is blamed, in part, on their tendency to trivialize women's problems—itself the product of gender stereotypes that construe women's complaints as frivolous and illusory. An absence of biomedical evidence, thus, intersects with gender ideology, each reaffirming the other.

Sally: It's because it is a bunch of women complaining that doctors think it's not real. If we were men they would take it serious.

Hannah: It's not just hysterical women. It's a real problem.

Morgan: In their [doctors] eyes, it looks like hysterical women so, rather than trying to figure this out, they call it a mental problem and give you a drug.

In practical terms, the cultural standard of dismissing, demeaning, and doubting women comes to shore up sufferer's claims that they have been wrongly labeled and treated. It also lends credibility to their moving from doctor to doctor in search of one willing to take women seriously. In certain regards, therefore, those who suffer from FMS are the inheritors of earlier political victories of the women's health movement, which in the 1970s critiqued the clinical power and authority of male-dominated medicine over women's bodies. Part of the solution, as articulated by 1970s feminists, was for women to refuse to be voiceless and passive objects of medical treatment and demand to be involved directly and actively in their own medical decision-making. Changes of this sort in childbirth practices and breast cancer treatment are two of the most dramatic and visible reforms attributable to the women's health movement (Morgen 2002; Olson 2002), but some of the general demands advanced by feminists three decades ago have become part of the general cultural fabric in which women today experience illness and disease.[3] As a case in point, it emboldens women patients to reject psychogenic interpretations of their health and search for health care providers less likely to trivialize their complaints.

Sufferers also counter psychogenic explanations by attempting rationally to resolve the epistemological crisis brought on by their illness. They persist in their effort to reconcile the deeply felt contradiction between a lack of biomedical evidence for their symptoms, and the certainty they

have about their own embodied distress. By confronting the epistemological crisis head on, they work through the question, "How do we know
what we know?" In the end, they answer by reaffirming the commonsense
attitude: being in their bodies allows *them* a privileged standpoint to assess the reality of their symptoms. Reasoning in terms of the mind-body
dualism, they assure themselves over and over that their symptoms are *in
their bodies* and, consequently, cannot be *in their minds*, whether medically
visible or not. Even as women have lost some of their conviction on this
score, to avert the total collapse of social reality they return time and again
to what seems manifestly apparent: truly embodied experiences *cannot* be
merely imaginary. The following remarks are illustrative of the common
claim that those who suffer, as a consequence of being in their bodies,
are the ultimate authorities when it comes to determining the validity of
their symptoms.

> **Alice:** Here they were telling me nothing is wrong, but *I knew* something
> was wrong. *I knew* this was something going on in my body.

> **Phyllis:** *I know* what it feels like for your body not to feel right. You don't
> feel good and something is wrong.

> **Sally:** We are in these bodies. *We know* what it feels like to have fibrofog, to
> be hurting all the time, to have all these symptoms.

Finally, and most compelling of all, these sufferers speak of the life-
changing effects of their illness as further evidence that their symptoms
are profoundly tangible, not simply imaginary. In other words, the impact
of their symptoms can be seen in the material world, thereby functioning
as a type of bitter validation that their symptoms undeniably exist. Doris,
Ellen, and Morgan each speak of the objective troubles brought on by
their illness.

> **Doris:** FMS is real. It changed my life.

> **Ellen:** This is a real disease that is debilitating. We are not hypochondriacs.
> We have real pain. We have real health problems. We are real people and
> we are sick. It totally changes your quality of life.

> **Morgan:** It's real all right. I mean why would anyone destroy their life on
> purpose? Why would I do that?

In sum, women sufferers attempt to resolve their own nagging uncertainties about the potential psychogenic basis of their illness by marshal-
ing evidence about the real character of their symptoms. Among other
things, as Morgan explains, their symptoms are real because their destructive consequences are beyond their volition. Ultimately, however, what
needs resolution is the contradiction set up by Valerie when she remarks,

"It's not a *mental* thing, it's something else. It is something *real.*" Culturally hemmed in by the mind-body distinction, sufferers define symptoms with psychological origins as illusory, whereas they experience their symptoms as categorically real. Consequently, either they defeat the psychogenic account of their illness or risk the dissolution of social reality altogether. The stakes of this battle are unimaginably high and the failure to recognize this would be to miss a central premise of the FMS story.

Conclusion

When the voice of the life world and the voice of medicine face off in the clinical context, the definition of reality is at stake. Drawing on taken-for-granted assumptions about reality, those who suffer "know" their illness to be "real." Biomedicine, however, negates women's commonsense reality. Trapped between two voices, two bodies of knowledge, and two realities, women sufferers avow their experience. In an effort to counter psychogenic accounts of their condition, they emphasize their overall mental well-being, the specific and secondary character of their psychological distress, the influence of gender bias in doctor–patient interactions, their epistemological advantage, and the undeniable material consequence of their symptoms. Although these techniques of self-assurance offer them a modicum of solace by holding the psychogenic account of their illness at bay, their distressing symptoms still lack *social* validation and meaning. Everyday reality is a social product, not a personal endeavor (Berger and Luckmann 1967). Accordingly, those who suffer must press on in search of a tool to rebuild the parameters of everyday life. That tool, and the focus of the next chapter, is a medical diagnosis in line with their convictions.

6

Diagnostic Transformations

n the same way that each account of fibromyalgia syndrome (FMS) includes the struggle to be understood, each account also includes a moment of transformation when the sufferer learns of the diagnosis and her suffering is finally acknowledged medically. It is hard to overstate the significance this event represents for most women. It is a ceremonial or ritual moment representing the passage from desperation and isolation to salvation. Laura and Emily provide typical descriptions of how it felt to have their condition diagnosed.

> **Laura:** Having someone finally listening who had an explanation. The doctor asked me questions that left my mouth hanging open. "How did you know that?" It was the most incredible relief. It was like being saved. By the time he was finished I knew that he could not have asked such good questions if I did not have something real. I am not hypochondriac. This is not all in my head. This has a name. Here is a man with all these credentials and it is real.

> **Emily:** I felt on top of the world. This thing that had been plaguing me for so many years finally had a name and it was real and here was this man who knew about it and can help me. I felt fabulous. I mean it was just like a reassurance that I'm not crazy when other doctors had been saying that for so long. It was a really good feeling.

This chapter describes women's transformations when finally hearing a diagnosis for their condition. As is the case for Laura and Emily, the moment of diagnosis holds pride of place in the narrative accounts of FMS sufferers. After a long period during which no one seemed to listen or to understand them, leaving them frightened, angry, and alienated, being diagnosed brings tremendous redemptive possibilities. Someone did understand them and that someone is an authoritative expert who can make sense of their illness within a logical framework of medical knowledge and, in so doing, endow it with order, meaning, and legitimacy. In brief, the name, "fibromyalgia," simultaneously certifies the suffering and the sufferer. All the while, it is hard to miss the gender dynamic in this process, seen clearly in Laura and Emily's recollection: the long ignored, misunderstood, and ill-treated woman, finally finds her savior who, by virtue of *his authority*, validates *her experience.*

Even as a diagnosis restores some parameters of sufferers' everyday lives, they quickly learn the limitations of the FMS diagnosis itself. Because FMS has no effective treatment, no objective test, and no definite origin, it remains marginalized and so do its sufferers. Consequently, they find themselves trapped between appealing to biomedical authority vis-à-vis their diagnosis, and the contested biomedical status of the diagnosis itself. What follows is a description of how women expectantly embrace their new diagnosis, while traversing its marginality, as they work to recreate boundaries of the self and everyday life.

The Diagnosing of Fibromyalgia Syndrome

Without prompting, the women offer detailed descriptions of the moment their condition was finally diagnosed as fibromyalgia.[1] They remember this particular medical encounter well and narrate the sequence of events leading up to the vindicating proclamation, "You have fibromyalgia." In most cases, the women had never heard the word fibromyalgia before their diagnosing practitioner uttered it and, in most cases, that diagnosing practitioner was a rheumatologist.[2] Yet, this new word, fibromyalgia, rapidly becomes a part of the sufferer's everyday lexicon and one onto which she grafts tremendous hope for the future.

There Is a Name for This

Among the most important aspects of being diagnosed is finally having a name for the problem. A name—such an ostensibly simple thing—and yet sufferers refer to it again and again as bringing them relief, respite, and sanctuary. Laura and Emily's comments presented at the start of this chapter convey this sentiment, as do the comments of many others.

> **Ellen:** I was relieved that I had a name to put on the symptoms and a name to put onto how I felt. I finally knew what was wrong with me then. It was a relief to know that.

Betsy: It was a great relief. It was so good to finally have a name to go with my problems.... That was the greatest thing to me, to have a name for why I feel this way all the time.

Ellen and Betsy's remarks specifically reveal the uneasiness that arises from experiences that cannot be named. The origins of this disquiet involve the link between naming and the social construction of reality. Recall from Chapter 1, Charles Rosenberg's somewhat polemical assertion that a disease does not exist until it is named. From medical clinicians who formally declare the existence of a new diagnosis, to the laity, who become familiar with the basics of new medical knowledge over time, a diagnostic name formally represents a social consensus about the existence of an illness. As seen in the following remarks, sufferers enthusiastically embrace the benefits of social consensus that a name implies.

Suzanne: It was like, finally, there is a name for this! This is not all in my head. I remember I cried when he [the doctor] told me. I said, "You mean it's not all a figment of my imagination? I'm not making myself feel this way?"

Wendy: The doctor said, "You have fibrositis." That is what he called fibromyalgia at the time. When he told me, I had a smile on my face. I'm not crazy, and there is honestly something wrong with me and there is a name for it.

Courtney: You're so extremely relieved to find that there is a name for all these awful things that have been going on in your body, and that you're not insane.

Margaret: My first reaction was relief, knowing that there is a name to it and you are not crazy.

The moment of diagnostic naming represents immediate psychological amnesty for women sufferers because a name makes *it* (their illness) a real *thing* and, therefore, is not the product of their imagination. In principle, language socially objectifies experience (Berger and Luckmann 1967: 68). Moreover, the moment of diagnostic naming also represents a sense of immediate relief because it gives sufferers a language in which to speak to others of their suffering. Wendy, Morgan, and Emily each recall making this important connection.

Wendy: It [being diagnosed] felt great because I finally had something I could tell people. I could say, "This is what is wrong with me." Instead of saying, "Well, I have this, and this, and this, and this, and nobody knows what is wrong with me."

Morgan: The day I was diagnosed, I called everyone on the phone and told them, "I have fibromyalgia!" It was strange but I was happy. I mean, these were people that had spent years listening to me complain, and now I had a name for my disease, not just a long list of complaints.

Emily: I feel more comfortable talking to people about it because I can say, "I have fibromyalgia" instead of saying "I have this thing that causes pain in my joints and no doctor will believe me." [Laughs] Now it's like, "Look, it's proven that this exists and this is what I have and here's what it's all about." So, I'm more comfortable talking about it. . . . I feel like I have been validated. I mean I don't know if others had a problem with it before or not but I certainly did. Not knowing if it's in my head, like people were saying, or how to explain it to people. Now I can say, "Its called fibromyalgia and if you want information, look on the Internet." Or, "Let me fax you this article on it so you know a little bit more about it."

Thus, having a diagnostic name organizes chaotic complaints that sufferers have endured for years but have been unable to convey meaningfully to others. To be sure, they find some comfort in being able to explain intelligibly their suffering, but the name represents far more than the ability to complain more coherently. Specifically, a diagnostic name holds the promise of reincorporating the sufferer into the social world from which she has been alienated.

Barbara: Before, I felt very alone. I didn't feel like I could talk to people about all of this, about all of the symptoms. . . . That's the biggest difference between before and after [the diagnosis]. Before, you're just aimlessly wandering around *feeling like an alien* wondering why you're feeling like you are. Afterwards, at least, you have a name.

Jessica: *You feel like an alien* because no one understands you. So you try not to talk about it because no one believes you anyway. When I was diagnosed, it made me feel less alien. After years of trying to explain to people what was wrong with me I was able to say, "I have fibromyalgia. It is a real thing with a real name that doctors believe in."

Barbara highlights feeling alone, being cut off, and lacking direction; Jessica emphasizes feeling incomprehensible and ultimately not believable. In both cases, however, the comments reveal the outsider status that results from a nameless experience and the inability to communicate that experience to others. Having a name for their experiences opens vistas for reestablishing social citizenship and it is essential to women's diagnostic transformations.

The Tender Point Examination

In addition to the importance of finally having a name for their illness, sufferers also stress the significance of finally having a test—a tender point examination—to prove that their illness really exists. Whether diagnosed by a rheumatologist, another specialist, or a general practitioner, each of the women in this study had a tender point examination as part of her diagnostic work-up. To remind the reader, FMS criteria include widespread pain for six or more months and tenderness in eleven of eighteen tender point locations pressed during a physical examination, with some flexibility in the number of positive tender points, depending on other clinical observations. The points are pressed with enough pressure to turn the examiner's fingernail white (approximately four kg) and the point is deemed positive if the patient confirms mild or greater tenderness in response.

Sufferers emphasize the value of finally having positive test results after the frustrating and extensive run of normal tests and examinations.

> **Cindy**: I'd seen tons of different rheumies [rheumatolgists] and they found nothing wrong. Every test was normal. But not this time. I was diagnosed by tender points. Dr. Peters did the test and said, "It's positive." Wow! That was a big deal!

In the eyes of sufferers, a positive tender point exam provides tangible evidence of their illness, and so it is hardly surprising that the women invoke the degree to which they fit, or in some cases surpass, the diagnostic requirements established by the American College of Rheumatology (ACR).[3]

> **Karen:** My doctor did a tender point exam and I had pretty much all of them.

> **Hannah:** They were doing the eighteen-point thing where if you have pain in those areas, then you have fibromyalgia. . . . I had just about every single one of them.

> **Wendy:** I went to the rheumatologist and he did the tender point exam. To be diagnosed, you have to have eleven of eighteen tender points. I had *more* than eighteen!

> **Doris:** The rheumatologist put me through the pressure point test and I responded to that. I think probably to all of them. It was a very definite diagnosis. The doctor was very definite.

As with others, Doris calls attention to the link between her unmistakable response to the tender point examination and her doctor's diagnostic certitude. As told by sufferers, from exacting, comprehensive, and arduous investigation, a certain and conclusive diagnosis emerged.

> **Laura:** He [the doctor] did an extensive interview, taking copious notes, and found that all the points with fibromyalgia were positive. He was definite. It was a positive diagnosis.

> **Emily:** He [the doctor] did a trigger point test and a very long history. He spent an hour and a half with me and he diagnosed me right there and he said, "There's no question you have fibromyalgia, I don't know what is going on here and why no one else has diagnosed it."

Time and again, sufferers assert that both their test results and their doctors were *very* positive in establishing the diagnosis of FMS. In fact, many explain that the results from their diagnostic examinations not only exceeded the standard requirements for a positive fibromyalgia diagnosis, but actually defined the very essence of the disease itself. For example, Suzanne and Ellen each report that their diagnosing physician identified them as a "classic case" of fibromyalgia because the specifics of their condition, including their tender point exam, fully epitomized the syndrome. Similarly, after her tender point examination, Cindy says that her rheumatologist told her she was a "textbook case." Sufferers underscore the degree to which their tender point examination left no room for diagnostic doubt or indecision. They have fibromyalgia. About this their doctors are certain.

As noted by Hugh Smythe in the early 1970s, the diagnostic utility of tender points lay in patients being unaware of them. As such, he argued that tender points provided a mechanism for distinguishing between bizarre forms of psychogenic rheumatism and the mundane, presumably organic, pain of FMS. Using a parallel logic, women draw attention to their lack of knowledge about tender points at the time of examination as robust evidence of the tangible, physical basis of their condition.

> **Margaret:** I had the tender point test when I was diagnosed. I didn't know what the rheumatologist was doing at the time, but, well, it hurt enough that he had to pull me down from the ceiling.

> **Jessica:** No one ever told me about tender points, but when the rheumatologist pressed on them, I wanted to come out of my skin. Every point was positive!

Embedded within sufferers' narration of their unambiguously positive tender point examination, especially given their original ignorance about such points, is a certain degree of self-satisfaction. In the abstract, it would seem that every patient should hope that his or her medical tests reveal nothing wrong. Negative results should be comforting. They give the individual permission to go on with his or her life, putting aside unsettling fears. But, as seen in the previous chapter, negative test results so contradict sufferers' subjective reality that they have precisely the opposite effect; they produce anxiety, not relief. Perhaps, then, we can appreciate women's seemingly peculiar satisfaction at being told that, in fact, *something* is wrong with them and that that something is captured in a positive tender point examination.

> **Suzanne:** It helped so much when I was diagnosed. It was really important to me.... There is *something*. There is the ACR diagnosis.

> **Morgan:** You have to have tender points to be diagnosed. There really is *something* wrong and doctors can prove It.

Women are relieved by their unequivocally positive tender point exams for good reason. After months or years without medical verification, a doctor's ability to translate their subjective reality via tender points represents a significant breakthrough. Like having a name, having a test makes their illness a real "thing" and, consequently, it makes them feel sane. It confirms women's sense of reality and their commonsense attitude that deeply felt bodily sensations, after all, are quintessentially valid.

The central place of the tender point examination in women's narrative accounts also reveals the cultural power of the objectifying biomedical gaze. Biomedical facts about the body, based on objectively determined standards generated through the accumulation of data, are culturally considered the final arbitrator in matters of embodiment. More specifically, biomedical facts about the physical body determine standards by which to distinguish the normal from the abnormal body and, in turn, legitimate diagnoses and therapeutic interventions. In sum, knowledge accumulated through biomedicine's objectifying techniques creates what Michel Foucault (1975) calls "bio-power"; it authorizes (or denies) the intervention of biomedicine into the body and lives of patients.

Foucault primarily addresses the negating aspects of bio-power, or how patient subjectivity is subverted (and reinterpreted) by the objectification techniques of biomedicine, resulting in biomedically informed social control. Even while this claim remains salient, another important aspect of biomedicine's current hegemony is the *affirming* aspect of bio-power, or the desire on the part of patients to have their subjectivity confirmed through biomedicine's techniques and to be granted the appropriate rights and privileges accordant to the sick role. Sufferers want their illness framed in orthodox biomedical terms. Leaving aside the problems with the tender point examination for now, in the eyes of sufferers, the existence of a medical test, its scientifically determined standards of normality and abnormality, and their unambiguously abnormal test results, represents a confirmation of their sense of reality and the existence of their condition. In short, sufferers' emphasis on the tender point examination demonstrates the culturally affirming qualities of bio-power.

Now I Know What I'm Dealing With

Having a diagnosis means sufferers have a real disease with a biomedical name and a biomedical test to prove it. In more practical terms, having a diagnosis means that sufferers now know what *it* is, and with that knowledge comes certain valuable gains. For example, in addition to confirming their sanity, the diagnosis also confirms that they are not dying. To their great relief, sufferers come to learn that FMS is a chronic, but not terminal, illness. As a result, the diagnosis brings some resolution of the dual anxieties that one must be either crazy or dying from an undetected disease.

> **Evelyn:** Well, I guess since I know what it is, I don't worry all the time about something being wrong. . . . Because you think it could be something life threatening, because you feel like you're dying.

> **Paula:** I knew that I was sick. I didn't know what I was sick with. I guess it was kind of good in some ways to know that I wasn't going to die because no one I knew got that sick without dying. In fact I expected to die a couple of times and I didn't. So, a relief from that.

> **Betsy:** It was awful before, because there were times when I thought it was terminal. Now that I know that this is something that I can survive, that it is not going to kill me, I love life again. I love the trees. I love the grass. I love the sunshine. I just love every day.

Knowing what *it* is also introduces sufferers to corresponding information about *it*, or a "knowledge environment" (Giddens 1991). A diagnosis "provides a sense that one is living in an orderly world" and "that one's condition can be located in medical indices and in libraries" (Hilbert 1984: 368). Such reassurance is welcome, given the extended period of self-doubt endured by sufferers. Knowing what *it* is also means that sufferers and their health care providers can draw on the available medical information about the condition. Clinicians and sufferers alike can turn to the medical indices and libraries to develop a practical plan of action.

> **Mary:** Now I know what I was dealing with, and so did the doctors. I looked it up in an old medical book. It really did help to know.

> **Courtney:** You're just so relieved that you know it is something. It means that people can dig in and deal with everything involved. I mean, until you know what it is, you just jump from here to there.

> **Barbara:** At least I had something to go on. I had something that I could research. I had something I could work with and try and modify. Before, it's like you feel like crap and that's all there is to it. Everything you're doing isn't helping. It doesn't matter how early you go to bed, and nothing seemed to help at all. So, with the diagnosis comes tools to make changes and to find improvements.

As seen in these remarks, having a diagnosis locates sufferers in a field of action and, consequently, facilitates their sense of agency. At least now, sufferers have "something to work with." They can, for example, go to a library, the Internet, or a bookstore, and read about their illness with an eye toward its future management. They can join or form an FMS support group and learn practical tips from others about how to cope with their symptoms. They can educate themselves, their own health care providers, their family members, and the general public about FMS. Having a diagnosis gives individual women access to educational and support resources and a restored feeling of efficacy after a sustained period of helplessness.

Yet, the "something to work with" conveyed to sufferers through the name, the positive tender point examination, and the vast medical and lay FMS knowledge environment, is infused with medical controversy. Critics argue that the name itself is a misnomer; the term fibromyalgia suggests a disorder in muscle or fibrous tissue when no such dysfunction has been found. By calling the collection of unexplainable symptoms fibromyalgia, critics contend, sufferers falsely assume they have a disease when their symptoms might more accurately be called diffuse suffering or chronic pain accompanied by a cluster of disagreeable symptoms (Block 1999; Bohr 1996; Ehrlich 2003). Likewise, the ACR criteria, including tender point counts, rely on the patient's subjective evaluation of pain, despite the veneer of objectivity it exemplifies to sufferers. Finally, the proliferation of FMS research has been attacked by some physicians as a professional campaign to promote an iatrogenic disease, whereas the lay community of patients with FMS is said to disseminate "goofy illness attributions" and a series of untested theories through the Internet and other venues (Bohr 1995; Hadler 1997a; Hadler 1997b).

Not all sufferers are aware of the specific reasons for the controversy surrounding their new diagnosis, but none of the women interviewed were unaware that controversy exists. For most, it does not take long before they find themselves peculiarly betwixt and between—neither healthy nor "diseased"—and they must confront the realities of this predicament in their everyday lives.

Limits of Diagnosis

Lack of Effective Treatment

The most immediate limitation to sufferers' newfound FMS diagnosis is its inability to translate into effective treatment. At the time of diagnosis, most sufferers are told that, although their condition is not fatal, it nonetheless responds poorly to medical interventions. Consequently, the sense of deliverance at the moment of diagnosis almost immediately butts up against the realization that having FMS portends a lifetime of chronic illness. Sufferers lament this unfortunate state of affairs, like Betsy, who notes: "It was a great thing to have a diagnosis but, unfortunately, they couldn't offer any treatment."

Part of what motivates sufferers to press on in a tenacious search for a diagnosis is the hope for a remedy for their condition. Ideally, a diagnosis charts a course of medical action and, in turn, a cure or palliative solution. But FMS is not an ideal diagnosis. Even though sufferers are greatly relieved to learn that their condition is not life threatening and motivated to learn more about it, the bleak prognosis is nevertheless discouraging.

> **Joyce:** After I was diagnosed, I went home and I looked it up on the [Inter]net and I went to the library. Within a week, I had a few inches' stack of information. I was not very thrilled. It can be debilitating. The first thing they tell you is that it does not go away. You would like to hear that you could do something to make it go away.

Consequently, the sense of relief that comes with a diagnosis is partly offset by learning that fibromyalgia is both debilitating and incurable. Accordingly, FMS sufferers articulate frustration and regret that so little can be done to alleviate their symptoms now that their illness is at last recognized as real. This frustration is both immediate and long term, as expressed by Suzanne and Robin, respectively.

> **Suzanne:** It was a relief that there was a name for it. Yet there was the doctor telling you that there's nothing you can do about it. So . . . it's like you've been sentenced. Sentenced is a strong word maybe. I knew it would not kill me. I knew it would not put me in a wheelchair, but you realize that you're gonna have to deal with the pain forever. There's no cure for this. So, on the one hand it was wonderful. On the other hand, it was, like, what do I do now?

> **Robin:** I thought maybe that, since they had a name for it, that they would be able to give me something that would help. That hasn't happened yet and that was eight years ago.

The collective results of years of FMS treatment research are manifest in the lives of the women in this study. In response to a collection of drug, physical, cognitive or behavioral, and alternative modalities, few appreciable gains have been made and, independent of treatment modality, many significant setbacks have occurred. As captured in the titles of dozens of research articles, the operative phrase is not the "treatment of FMS" but rather the "management of FMS." Even this language grossly distorts clinicians' ability to control the enigmatic ebb and flow in symptomology. The ability even to manage FMS symptoms medically is, without question, highly limited. Consequently, the FMS diagnosis is experienced as dispiriting. The grim prognosis forces sufferers to abandon the dream of health and carry in its stead the near certainty of a future constrained by sickness. Nevertheless, with a name for their condition and a restored sense of self-confidence and efficacy, sufferers pick themselves up and search for whatever modest improvements modern medicine might afford them.

Medical Skepticism and Other Barriers to Quality Care

Those who suffer from FMS unknowingly enter a divided clinical world. At first, they feel reassured to have a diagnosis and imagine that it will serve them well as they seek out medical assistance for what they now know to be their chronic FMS symptoms. But, with their new diagnosis in hand, sufferers run headlong into a lukewarm or hostile reception from most rank-and-file physicians. Some physicians believe in FMS and provide care for its sufferers on the basis of that diagnosis, but many do not. For these reasons, having a diagnosis rarely ends the sequence of medical encounters in which sufferers find both their symptoms and themselves suspect. In general, having an FMS diagnosis does little to lessen their struggle with doctors and other health care providers who remain predisposed to framing their illness as emotional or mental rather than physical.

> **Wendy:** When doctors find out you have fibromyalgia, they think you're a hypochondriac. Yeah, I'm a hypochondriac. I have nothing better to do with my time or my money than go from doctor to doctor.

> **Rachel:** I went to the emergency room recently and the doctor—two sentences after I said the word "fibromyalgia"—he leaned over and said, "I notice that you're a very nervous person." I wanted to slap his face. As soon as I said "fibromyalgia" he assumed I had a mental problem. He was saying "two plus two equals seven."

> **Suzanne:** I do *not* have a mental illness! ... There are some people in the medical field that still believe that it [fibromyalgia] is a mental thing. It's like coming up against a brick wall again and again.

As told by sufferers, they customarily encounter doctors who reject a biophysical interpretation of FMS. Some physicians do so by directly or indirectly conveying their sense that FMS is something of a fashionable diagnosis for underlying mental illness, whereas others attack the credibility of the diagnosis itself. The following remarks are just some of the many that capture the discordance these encounters represent to sufferers and the anger they evoke.

> **Evelyn:** Most of them [doctors] say, "Oh, a doctor just gave you that diagnosis so you think you have something." One doctor told me that there really

is no such thing as fibromyalgia and that they just made that diagnosis up. I was angry.

Wendy: Many doctors still, to this day—because FMS is a syndrome, not a disease—don't believe in fibromyalgia because there are no laboratory tests that prove it. It is hard to find a doctor. When I interviewed my doctor, I asked her if she believed in fibromyalgia. Why would you go to a doctor who thinks you are a hypochondriac, who thinks you are a liar, who thinks you are nuts?

As with Wendy, sufferers refuse to see doctors who suggest they are intentionally or unintentionally exaggerating their symptoms. Yet, given the widespread medical disparagement of FMS, this makes finding health care providers who believe in the disorder and who are willing to care for its sufferers—referred to as "fibro-friendly"—an ongoing dilemma and a top priority. The ordinary course of action involves moving from doctor to doctor as the provider makes his or her critical stance toward FMS known during the clinical encounter.

Cindy: You spend a lot of your time just looking for fibro-friendly doctors. You might find one that's okay for a while, but then he starts having less patience with all the symptoms. After a while, you have to start over again [and get a new doctor].

Ellen: Folks with fibromyalgia run into problems with doctors. There are a lot of doctors who don't treat it. There are a lot of doctors who don't know anything about it. Then, there are the doctors who do know about it but don't believe in it. You don't get a lot of good treatment out there. I have gone through a lot of doctors. Since then [the six years since diagnosis], I have gone through ten doctors. It is a nightmare for people with fibromyalgia because it is not considered a debilitating disease, but we all know from experience that it is. It is debilitating and disabling. It is really frustrating what these doctors put you through.

Many patients with FMS, thus, encounter considerable obstacles to quality and sympathetic care and, once again, they cycle rapidly through doctors, effectively finding their post-diagnosis medical encounters to differ little, if at all, from those before diagnosis.

The problem in finding a fibro-friendly provider is straightforward: there simply are not enough of them to care for the large number of FMS sufferers. One of the women in this study, a local FMS and CFS support group leader, conducted an interesting survey in her small town that illustrates the predicament patients with FMS and CFS face. There are no rheumatologists in her small town but she sent a survey to all forty-five general practitioners in her community, asking them if they believed in fibromyalgia and chronic fatigue syndrome and if they would treat patients with these disorders. Of the thirty-eight physicians responding to her survey, thirteen, or approximately one third, said they believed in the disorder, but only four said they would treat those who suffer from it. In practical terms, this means that more than eighty members of her local support group, as well as an unknown number of others suffering from FMS or CFS not affiliated with the group, are restricted to only four of the forty-five local primary care providers.

Although discouraging, this survey at least provided local support group members with helpful information. In general, the FMS support community provides a host of resources to aid sufferers in the difficult search for sympathetic providers. Many local support group leaders compile and keep active lists of supportive doctors in their communities. Several national organizations compile lists as well, often working with information they receive from local groups to generate lists that can be accessed online or requested through the mail. Because these formal lists increase the chances of receiving compassionate care, they are widely used. Moreover, the informal comparing and contrasting of providers is standard fare among support group members. Within real and virtual support groups, women routinely share the names of physicians who have given them sympathetic care and warn of those to avoid. The FMS support community also provides other tools through its support groups, self-help books, newsletters, and Web sites, such as instructions for interviewing doctors to determine their stance on FMS before establishing a doctor-patient relationship.

The existence of a formal and informal network of information exchange has led some detractors of the diagnosis to assert that sufferers simply shop for sympathetic doctors to avoid any and all medical criticism of FMS (Bohr 1996). This accusation is hard to deflect, given the "how-to" resources generated by the FMS support community for selecting a fibro-friendly doctor and the frequency with which most patients move from doctor to doctor in search of sympathetic care. Although critics see this as a damning indictment, patients simply cannot imagine doing otherwise. To repeat Wendy's earlier comment: "Why would you go to a doctor who thinks you are a hypochondriac, who thinks you are a liar, who thinks you are nuts?" The concerns of detractors aside, such a doctor-patient relationship is unsustainable.

Whereas the relative scarcity of providers sympathetic to the FMS diagnosis represents the central barrier to quality care, the problems associated with managing fibromyalgia patients also have an undermining effect. Even sufferers understand that they are "difficult patients," which further restricts their ability to find and keep sympathetic doctors. Patients with FMS can easily burn out even supportive doctors with the sheer number of their chronic complaints. They know also that their medical management is complex and their improvement likely to be negligible. They understand at an experiential level what research consistently demonstrates: physicians find patients with chronic somatic complaints that show little improvement with therapeutic intervention frustrating and, when possible, they try to minimize their contact with such patients (Mechanic 1992).

Patients with FMS also know that they take a lot of consultation time in a health care environment where time is scarce. Wendy and Morgan sketch out these problems as it relates to their own care and the care of patients with FMS, generally.

> **Wendy:** If doctors can't give you a pill or cut on you, then they don't have a clue. They have no idea what to do with us. We are difficult patients. We don't go in with one thing wrong with us. We go in with a list. You write them all down, too, because you can't remember them anyway. You need to have an extended appointment. We are not talking fifteen minutes. It takes forty-five minutes. They think you are a pain in the ass.... You need to find a doctor that will take the time to work with you.

> **Morgan:** I don't blame the doctors really. I mean, we take so much time. When I go to the doctor I have a long list of all the things that have been bugging me since my last appointment. I think treating fibromyalgia patients is hard and nothing they do makes us that much better.

Patients with FMS take a lot of time with the doctor, and all the time in world, at best, yields only modest gains. Not surprisingly, a simple cost-benefit analysis puts the institutional squeeze on patients with FMS. All the existing professional disincentives for dealing with such problematic patients are heightened in managed care organizations (MCO) that currently dominate the U.S. health care system (Ellis 1998; Robinson 1999). All of the women in this study were insured through either a public or private managed care organization,[4] and stories about barriers to health care visits, providers, referrals, and services were the norm.

> **Paula:** I'm currently in an HMO and I'm having a real hard time finding good care.... And I'm now in the same position as every other frigging fibromyalgia patient in town is in and that is looking for a doctor that will treat me decently with my insurance. Gosh what fun!

> **Sally:** HMOs, along with SSA [Social Security Administration], are part of the Evil Empire. You have to battle for the care you need.

> **Alice:** In the state's health plan there are things that will be paid for and things that will not.... The waiting list to see rheumatologists is five weeks. Doctors are limited by what insurance will pay and what they won't. And

that tells the doctor what he should order and what he should not. New things like PET scans [positron emission tomography scans] to see if there's a dysfunctional brain, most insurance will not pay for that. So, while I can't blame doctors, I don't feel like many of them try to help us.

Despite all these difficulties, a few women have found providers who take them and their complaints seriously. In these rare cases, women unmistakably express their appreciation for finally having a sympathetic ear. For example, Courtney uses a religious metaphor to convey the significance of getting supportive care.

Courtney: I have finally found a good doctor, a rheumatologist. It was like getting to Mecca after two and a half years of searching for a doctor who even knew what I was talking about, . . . someone who didn't treat me like I was a woman who didn't have anything better to do than go to the doctor.

Courtney's remarks, again, draw attention to the tendency for gender stereotypes to fill the gap of medical uncertainty and to women's sense that part of the struggle for quality health care involves overcoming such stereotypes. In a similar vein, Joyce explains how her successful search for quality care meant finding someone with an interest in listening to women and the time to do so—qualities she suggests are rare among physicians as a result of organizational dictates and the character of their medical practice.

Joyce: I discovered that I did much better with a nurse practitioner than with doctors. I was in an HMO and I had changed doctors about a half dozen times. I finally found somebody who was interested in women and interested in listening to me. I did not do well with physicians, male or female, because they just don't have the time. Nurse practitioners are willing to take the time, research it with you and say, "Let's see if this works or not." The physicians say, "Take this pill. See you."

Finally, some of the difficulties related to finding and keeping a sympathetic provider are the result of the constantly changing health care insurance landscape (Emanuel and Dubler 1995; *States of Health* 1996). As insurers and providers merge, consolidate, and otherwise restructure, Americans, in general, are moved in and out of different health insurance arrangements as their employers' shop for the least expensive benefits package. Similarly, patients covered by state or federal health programs find their benefits have atrophied during recent years and that some providers are (or become) unwilling to treat the publicly insured (or treat very many of the publicly insured) on grounds that they bring below-market compensation. These factors undermine the ability of many of us to find quality health care and ensure its continuity; given the barriers patients with FMS already face in this regard, the burden is especially hard felt. For example, sufferers explain how their hard-won efforts to find good providers and develop good working relationships with them, although rare, can be lost in an instant when they lose insured access to that provider.

It is the exception to find an FMS sufferer who favorably evaluates her medical care in the wake of her diagnosis. More commonly, her complaints focus on the lack of effective treatments, widespread medical disparagement of the FMS diagnosis, the scarcity of sympathetic physicians, and the inability or unwillingness on the part of physicians to manage the difficult FMS patient population. This goes a long way to explaining FMS sufferers' active use of complementary and alternative health care services (Berman and Swyers 1999; Crofford and Appleton 2001). Individuals diagnosed with fibromyalgia make significantly greater use of these services than patients with other rheumatic conditions, who themselves have higher than average utilization rates (Pioro-Boissett et al. 1996). Some research suggests that almost 90 percent of those diagnosed with FMS used some alternative care—a figure in line with reports from women in this study. Their eager consumption of goods and services from the alternative medical marketplace reveals, in part, their level of disaffection with medical orthodoxy.

The Other Side of the Doctor-Patient Interaction

The same cautionary statement must be made with respect to the validity of women's descriptions of their post-diagnosis medical encounters as was made about their pre-diagnostic encounters. Namely, they tell only *their* side of the story. Again, however, their comments can be interpreted in the context of findings from other studies—in this case, studies that show how physicians respond to the FMS diagnosis (or to related diagnoses such as CFS) and to patients so diagnosed. As already noted, many physicians find little reward in dealing with patients with medically unexplainable complaints. It is frustrating work and physicians' uncertainty about how to manage such patients can lead them to trivialize patients' complaints (Mechanic 1992). These general findings predictably translate to the case of FMS.

Based on interviews with Swedish physicians, Pia Asbring and Anna-Liisa Narvanen (2003) found that most are skeptical of CFS and FMS because they are illness, not disease, states. Indeed, they wonder if they are the right professionals to be dealing with such sufferers, and suggest that psychologists and social workers might be better suited to handle the everyday difficulties sufferers face. They also believe that patients with CFS or FMS tend to exaggerate their symptoms and should learn to live with them by developing better coping skills. Instead of coping well with common symptoms, physicians suggest these patients are "illness-fixated": they become convinced they are seriously physically ill, vigorously reject any suggestions to the contrary, actively seek out information about their condition, and over utilize health services. Quoting one of the physicians in the study:

> You see them, as a doctor, as very, very troublesome. They...I don't know...You find them to be querulous. They complain in expressive ways for long moments. They are fixed on themselves....Yes, I suppose they have a somewhat special personality (Asbring and Narvanen 2003: 715).

At least, according to the editor of the *Journal of Rheumatology*, Duncan Gordon (2003: 1665), rheumatologists in the United States feel similarly:

> In recent years I have also observed that many physicians express frustration directed not only at the FM construct, but also at the patient. This hostility seems related to the fact that patients with FM display very much more psychological distress than other patients. All this is further compounded by the lack of effective treatment for it and the fact that many patients have a record of adversarial interactions with the health care system. It is not surprising that some rheumatologists will not see patients that are referred to them for FM and others will only see the patient for a one-time assessment to exclude other conditions, but not provide ongoing care.

Research also shows that many physicians avoid diagnosing patients with CFS or FMS in the first place, fearing that they will become illness-fixated and that the label will ultimately become disabling (Asbring and Narvanen 2003; Barsky and Borus 1999; Broom and Woodward 1996). This strategy is a mix of paternalism and sense of professional duty to patients. Physicians also feel a professional obligation to meet the expectations of suffering patients in search of a diagnosis, which, in turn, can put them in a difficult situation with respect to applying controversial diagnoses (Broom and Woodward 1996; Hellström et al. 1998). For example, Dorothy Broom and Roslyn Woodward studied a small sample of Australian physicians and found that, whereas most are skeptical or cautious about the CFS diagnosis, some nevertheless felt that they could work with patients constructively to medicalize their problems under the auspices of the CFS diagnosis.

Moreover, when it comes to contested diagnoses, physicians and patients have very different operating assumptions. Jonathan Banks and Lindsay Prior's (2001) study of patient–doctor interactions in a CFS outpatient clinic in the United Kingdom is instructive. In brief, they found that patients with CFS, far more than physicians, fetishize biomedical orthodoxy. Doctors are not that concerned with finding a discrete biomedical sign for CFS and, instead, are willing to bend biomedicine's orientation to include the complexity of sufferers' illness through such means as the biopsychosocial perspective. Patients, conversely, see such efforts as derisive and push to have their illness located exclusively within a natural science framework. In short, patients frame their illness within a rigid biomedical disease model, but their physicians do not. In a study comparing patient and physician views about CFS Judith Richman and Leonard Jason (2001) reached a similar conclusion.

Needless to say, the different interests and assumptions of patients and physicians can result in conflicts when it comes to contested illnesses, conflicts that are likely to underlie the medical encounters described by FMS sufferers in this study. In practice, women's sense of being dismissed by doctors, in part, is the outcome of fundamentally different assumptions held by the two parties. Patients think of fibromyalgia as a disease, but physicians do not; patients think of tender points as objective evidence, but physicians do not; and patients favor organic explanations for their fibromyalgia, but physicians do not. When these two competing conceptual frameworks face off in the clinic, patients understandably feel invalidated and defensive.

Lay (Public) Invisibility

Unfortunately for beleaguered patients, the lay public also places little value on the FMS diagnosis. Taking its cue from medical experts, the general public approaches FMS and its sufferers with distrust. Most sufferers come across public cynicism toward the diagnosis and, as with medical criticism, public disparagement has corrosive consequences that can squander a sufferer's early enthusiasm about having a diagnosis. Valerie and Suzanne, for example, portray the disapproving response they received when they told people they had fibromyalgia.

> **Valerie:** Initially, I felt relieved to have a name because not knowing makes you feel like it's all in your head. But when I told people the name, the response of other people was a real downer. "That means they don't know what's wrong with you." "That's a wastebasket term." "Oh, everybody's got that." These types of things really put me under the table really fast. It is not an acceptable condition. It's okay to have cancer. You can get support, but it's not okay to get fibromyalgia. I find this very frustrating, and it makes me very angry.

> **Suzanne:** Someone will say, "Oh yeah, that's the nineties' disease." Or, "Everybody I know has that. That just means they can't diagnose you so they just tell you have fibromyalgia." It's like, here we go again.

What is more, the expert skepticism that trickles down to the laity is bolstered by commonsense skepticism. Not only do FMS sufferers appear entirely healthy as seen through biomedicine's gaze, but they also appear healthy to lay observers. Hannah summarizes the interplay of medical and lay invisibility with medical and lay skepticism.

Hannah: I really think that in many ways the sociological implications of fibromyalgia can almost be as debilitating as the physical, because of people's reactions to it.... It's hard when the doctors themselves don't even recognize it as a legitimate disease. In turn, your family and society at large approach you with skepticism too. So it's not only the doctors. Your own family thinks stuff like, "Oh my gosh, she's really going around the bend."... I think my family suffered an awful lot because I was really miserable and they thought I was nuts because there's no visible signs that you're sick. They thought I was making it up, I think. It put a real strain on my family relations.

Many recognized diseases are invisible to laity, but those afflicted are not approached with skepticism. For example, many forms of cancer remain invisible to the public, but medical verification of their existence converts into widespread public recognition of, and empathy for, cancer victims. Moreover, many forms of cancer (as well as other publicly invisible illnesses) become visible in the most dramatic fashion possible: they decompose the body and eventually result in death. In contrast, FMS clings to a marginal medical status and poses no current or future threat to the visible body or to the lives of sufferers. FMS does not summon a ready-made collection of cultural images of the blameless sufferer who, despite her tenacious struggle, eventually succumbs to the ravages of her disease. It does not hold a place in our individual or cultural fears, nor does it evoke individual or cultural compassion.

What is crucial about the lay invisibility of FMS is that it confirms, rather than disconfirms, the biomedical invisibility of the illness. Consequently, sufferers endure lay accusations that their complaints are evidence of mental illness or malingering. In effect, relationships and social interactions are constantly burdened by the sufferers' appearance of well-being. The phrases "But you look good" and "But you don't look sick" are ones that every FMS sufferer detests (see Figure 6.1). Accordingly, the support community produces articles, T-shirts, buttons, and posters that speak to the incongruity of private symptoms and public appearance with titles and logos such as "I don't feel as good as I look," "Seeing is not believing," and the like. Betsy sums up the frustrations of many sufferers when she notes, "All of a sudden you would really just rather look like shit and feel great!"

At home, in the workplace, and in larger social circles, sufferers find the public invisibility of fibromyalgia socially distressing. Without any

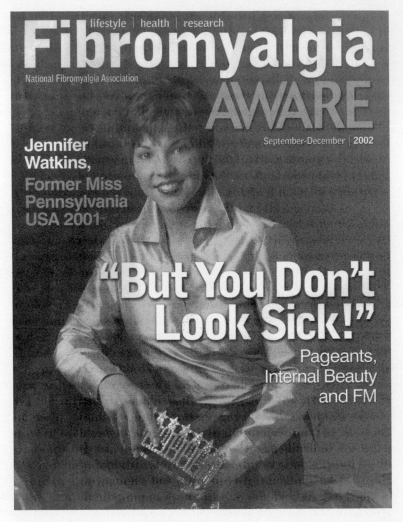

Figure 6.1   "But You Don't Look Sick!" Used by permission of the National Fibromyalgia Association.

visible explanation for their shortcomings, they routinely let down family and friends, and employers and coworkers grow frustrated with their poor and unpredictable performance. Betsy recently dropped from full time to part time in her position as a secretary for a large industrial firm. She finds that coming in late in the morning and leaving early in the afternoon greatly improves her symptoms, but she hates that coworkers interpret her restricted schedule as evidence of laziness in light of her outward appearance of good health. Others similarly lament how, when falling short of social expectations, they are left to bear the weight of social judgments they feel fundamentally misrepresent who they are.

Cindy: Your family gets angry because you can't do anything even though you look perfectly fine. People call this the invisible disease. It sure is invisible.... It makes me feel like I am lazy even though I know I am not.

Alice: Most of the time I look healthy. When they started calling this the invisible disease, that's basically what this is. It doesn't show. We tried so hard to prove that we are not complainers, that we are not crazy, that we are not stupid, that we are not lazy, that we are not trying to not help ourselves. That's a real inner struggle.... I don't really, but sometimes I wish I had an outward symptom that showed.

At least some outward symptom would help others understand their situation, explain their physical limitations, and absolve them of their failure to meet social demands. Instead, the moral character of the fibromyalgia sufferer is routinely called into question. In most cases, the sufferer turns public judgment in on herself and it becomes a real "inner struggle" to deflect, rather than internalize, the negative interpretations projected by others in countless daily interactions.

An outward sign of illness might also produce more public sympathy for FMS sufferers' requests for special reparations. After all, if they appear entirely normal, why should employers make special accommodations on their behalf or why should they receive public or private disability benefits and compensation? Negotiating the lack of public sympathy and assistance is a heavy burden associated with the invisibility of FMS.

Ellen: This disease is on the inside of our bodies, not the outside of our bodies. So people will look at us and say, "You don't look disabled." But we are, and they don't understand that. That makes it really hard for us to get disability [insurance], even though we are disabled.

Alice: I think if we were given a two-, three-, or four-hour time block to work, we might be able to make the effort if an employer was willing to believe in us. It annoys me sometimes when I hear that companies will do this for someone with cerebral palsy, Down syndrome, or multiple sclerosis, but we don't have a visible disability. That seems unfair. But that is the way those of us with FMS have to live.

Morgan: I hate that people give me the evil eye when I use disability parking at the mall. They look at me like: "You look pretty young and healthy." Or, "Looks like you could use some exercise," you know, because I could stand to lose some weight. I hate that kind of judgment because it makes you feel bad about yourself even though I know that without the sticker I can't do half the things I can do with it.

Marginal Medicalization

On one hand, women find the moment of diagnosis, with its name, its test, and its knowledge environment, dramatically self-affirming. On the other hand, they often feel defeated in knowing their illness is effectively untreatable and disparaged by the biomedical and lay communities. Despite this tension, none of the sufferers would trade their problematic diagnosis for the nightmare of no diagnosis at all. Jessica succinctly expresses this sentiment: "It's bad to have fibro, but it is worse to have it and not know it." Maude conveys a similar sentiment as she recalls rejecting condolences after telling someone about her recent FMS diagnosis: "Someone said to me, 'Oh, I am so sorry you have fibromyalgia. I have a friend that has that.' I said, 'I am so delighted to know I have it.'"

Nevertheless, a few sufferers entertain misgivings about the FMS diagnosis. For example, Barbara wonders what the current popularity of FMS might imply about the accuracy of her own diagnosis.

> **Barbara:** I had never heard of it, then once I got the diagnosis, it seemed like everybody has it. I have a really good friend who was just recently diagnosed by her chiropractor. I think it is really being overdiagnosed right now. I think it is kind of a "catch all" for any ailment that you might have. I really think it is being overdiagnosed, and that makes me wonder if I am one of those people who has a false diagnosis. I don't know.

Similarly, Hannah recalls telling a friend about having a tender point examination and the resultant questioning it evoked.

> **Hannah:** I was telling somebody else about how they diagnose it, and she said, "Well, those are all areas where anybody who is experiencing stress or works too hard or doesn't get enough sleep has pain anyway." That's for sure, so what is this? Some stupid disease. Who knows if it exists or it doesn't? . . . There isn't a test you can do that tells you that something is definitely wrong. . . . It's kind of a phony diagnosis, it really is.

Most sufferers, however, do not share such misgivings and even Barbara and Hannah merely raise, rather than embrace, them. Instead, most cling unwaveringly to the claim that fibromyalgia is an organic disease whose pathogenesis simply remains invisible. It is for this reason that many sufferers call FMS "the invisible disease." This is an interesting appropriation of the far more common contemporary use of this phrase to describe depression. Beginning several decades ago, mental health advocates, including the National Alliance for the Mentally Ill (NAMI), started calling depression "the invisible disease" as a political strategy to destigmatize mental illness through medicalization. Advocates claim that most mental illnesses, including depression, are organic brain disorders and, as legitimate physical disorders, they should be met with medical treatment, not social stigma.

The adoption by FMS sufferers of the phrase *invisible disease,* which appears in many popular FMS self-help books and resources, seems peculiar, given the hostility most have toward any suggestion equating FMS with depression. But the widespread use of this phrase, despite its pejorative connection to depression, reveals just how important biomedical and lay invisibility is to the FMS illness experience. Moreover, the same political gains that motivate mental health advocates—destigmatizing through medicalizing—spur on FMS sufferers and advocates as well, most of whom are familiar with, and embrace, a neurobiological account of FMS as a central nervous system disorder. For example, Alice explains: "Something in our brains is malfunctioning; it's saying okay attack your own body." As Suzanne remarks "Well it turns out that FMS *is* all in our heads, it's in our brains." Hannah explains: "There's interesting things coming out about this 'substance P' in the spinal fluid—that it actually carries and magnifies the pain message more than the average person."

Reciting promising research concerning organic abnormalities, sufferers assume it is only a matter of time until biomedicine lifts the veil of ignorance that plagues them. They anticipate a day when a clear-cut diagnostic test will silence the medical and lay skeptics alike. Indisputable verification, they believe, will finally bring to an end the remnants of self-doubt and public skepticism, provide the basis for public sympathy and compassion, and potentially validate claims on critical resources.

> **Barbara:** They need to find a way to test for this. They need to keep doing research looking for that, and they are. Doctors are finding levels of things within the body of an FMS person that are different than the body of a normal person. They are noticing that there are major differences, and once they can test it and can say for a fact that you do or you don't have it, then I think a lot of that hypochondriac thing will go away.

> **Sally:** It is a very real syndrome. Pain signals are not the only thing messed up in our nervous system. Lots of things are not working. I believe this is a nervous system disease. That is what causes the IBS and asthma. All of these have been stigmatized as psychosomatic. But they will figure this all out. Our brains are misfiring and it causes all these failures. But we might just have to hold out until they finally have a blood test or something. Then people will feel sorry for us. Then people will stop calling us crazy and all our symptoms psychosomatic. Maybe I will even get the disability [insurance] I deserve.

Gender, Self, and Diagnostic Transformations

Among the many consequences of what has been called "incomplete medicalization" by Broom and Woodward (1996) is a genuine threat to selfhood. For this reason, it should hardly be surprising that patients with

FMS become "intensively involved in efforts to get their self-images as ill persons confirmed" (Hellström et al. 1999: 11). Whereas critics suggest that patients' fixation on proving that they are genuinely ill undercuts the possibility of getting better (Hadler 1996), it seems evident, from the women in this study, that the benefits of diagnosis to one's overall sense of well-being are invaluable. The studies cited above, including Broom and Woodward (1996) and Helleström and colleagues (1999), also confirm these subjective benefits of diagnosis. Consequently, if we take the word of sufferers themselves, the verdict is clear: having a diagnosis dramatically improves patients' subsequent sense of well-being.

This is not to say that the FMS sufferers have a high level of well-being in the wake of their diagnosis; their lives are highly restricted and biomedicine has precious little to offer them. The subjectively reported quality of life for FMS sufferers is worse than that of sufferers of conditions that are widely recognized as seriously disabling (e.g., osteoarthritis, rheumatoid arthritis) and so, too, is their prognosis (Burckhardt et al. 1993). It would be misguided to hold the diagnosis itself responsible for these negative outcomes. From a patient perspective, well-being is considerably advanced by diagnosis and, because well-being, by definition, is subjective, patient subjectivity must be given serious weight. This line of reasoning seems all the more credible, given that no objective evidence indicates that the health status of FMS sufferers deteriorates after diagnosis (White et al. 2002).

My primary intent, however, is not to engage in the debate concerning the enabling or disabling character of FMS. Instead, the aim of this chapter is to explore the phenomenological consequences of the diagnosis, or how the *idea* of FMS shapes the experience of self and sickness, and why the idea has particular salience for women sufferers. With respect to these questions, applying the diagnostic classification of FMS to a woman sufferer changes the way she experiences herself. She becomes aware of her self in relationship to a diagnosis that confirms her sense of reality and brings order and meaning to otherwise chaotic and pointless suffering. The diagnosis effectively offers a redemptive passageway from one status to another: from the ashes of dubious and meaningless suffering emerges the vindicated and pro-active FMS sufferer. Having a diagnosis, to borrow the language Erving Goffman, initiates the FMS sufferer's "moral career," or the sequence of changes that a person passes through in his or her self-awareness and self-development (Goffman 1961: 128). Once diagnosed, the patient faces a new set of social encounters and experiences as an FMS sufferer, experiences she now shares with others who share her new social status. In the process, an intellectual construct developed by rheumatologists (the idea of FMS) reifies her illness itself;

she apprehends what is a product of human activity as if it is a fact of nature (Berger and Luckmann 1967: 89). The gender dynamics at the heart of these phenomenological consequences of diagnostic transformation are a crucial piece of the FMS story and one that requires further explication.

The Diagnostic Experiences of Men

Although the intentional focus of this study is *women* with FMS, four men diagnosed with the disorder were interviewed and occasional reference has been made to their experiences in endnotes throughout the text. To pursue the issue of gender as it relates to the FMS diagnostic transformation, a few comments are required here about men's markedly different responses to the experience of being diagnosed. At the same time, of course, we must proceed with caution about extrapolating from so few cases. This is a purely speculative venture and one that future research must address.

The key distinction in the men's diagnostic experience is that, unlike the women, they found little or no comfort in finally having a diagnostic name. Note the sharp dissimilarity between these comments and those of women sufferers presented earlier in the chapter.

Bruce: I heard people say, "It was a relief, something I could put a name on." That had no impact on me. That is not an important issue to me. What was important to me was how I was going to work with this.

Mark: At the time [of diagnosis] it was like, what do I do with this? They didn't even explain the word or that it was a multiple problem. They just said, "Here's a name for it and here's some more prescriptions."

Larry: Being diagnosed was a huge disappointment. I had been searching for an answer for so long and all I got was a brochure with a big meaningless word on it. The doctor didn't have anything to offer me and the brochure was depressing as hell. Basically, it just said eat a little better, get a little exercise, and maybe you will have a little less pain.

Scott: It [having a diagnosis] gives you some control, and everything in my life was out of control. I already knew. I had read fibromyalgia and chronic fatigue books. What else could it be? I was just ready to move on. Having someone with a degree on the wall finally say, "Yes, this is fibromyalgia," that was a relief. Now we can do the next step. . . . After I came back from the doctor, I cried. I was so relieved that finally I had the ear of someone who maybe knew what I was going through. He didn't seem to be either patronizing me, or making something up so he didn't have to deal with me and [could] get on to the next patient. And [the doctor] had a plan of action. I felt cared for . . . for the first time.

All four men had *pragmatic* responses to their diagnosis. Bruce directly notes that naming the disorder offered him no practical advantage, a point indirectly reiterated by both Mark and Larry. These three men found the diagnosis either unhelpful or disappointing. Scott's description is different in its emotiveness; being diagnosed made him feel thankful, understood, and cared for. Scott's remarks, thus, capture some of the same themes present in women's diagnostic transformations. Even so, having a diagnosis did not affirm Scott's sanity, his selfhood, or the reality of his illness. Already confident that he had fibromyalgia, he was merely waiting for an authority to confirm his self-diagnosis so he could "move on." One might, therefore, say that Scott did not benefit from the FMS diagnosis in and of itself, but rather from the compassion and empathy it represented, as well as the hope that a more proactive response to his condition might be forthcoming.

Many of the women also had pragmatic responses to their diagnosis. Recall that many asked themselves variants of the question: "How do I deal with this now that I know what it is?" But, for the women, "knowing what it is" is accompanied by a sense of self-affirmation absent in the responses from men. Likewise, all four men I interviewed had a tender point examination as part of their diagnostic work-up, but none of them raised its significance in terms of confirming their subjective reality or their physicians' diagnostic certitude. Larry unceremoniously recalls; "He [the doctor] asked questions and did the test and told me I had fibromyalgia." Bruce indifferently notes: "Yeah, he [the doctor] did a pressure point exam. He asked me about my sleep. He wasn't positive that I had it but it looked like it to him." Overall, the significance that a biomedical name and test represents for its ability to make symptoms real and sufferers feel sane is a pervading theme in the women's diagnostic experiences but missing from the men's.

One possible explanation for this difference could be that women searched longer for an answer for their symptoms than men and, thus, felt a greater sense of relief when their symptoms finally had biomedical representation via a diagnostic name and test. In fact, this is not the case. The average number of years from acute symptom onset to diagnosis for women in this sample was six and a half years. Two of the men spent less time in search of a diagnosis than this average but two spent significantly longer; the length of time from acute symptoms to diagnosis was three years for Bruce, six years for Larry, ten for Mark, and seventeen for Scott.[5] In general, it is likely true that the longer the search for diagnosis, the more comfort and reassurance diagnosis brings (Scott's case is illustrative), but gender difference in the duration of diagnostic search, at least in these few cases, does not account for women's greater sense of self-restoration after diagnosis. It is worth noting that it seems likely that men, on average, would have a longer road to diagnosis. Most practitioners understand that FMS primarily affects women, and, accordingly, this impacts their readiness to confirm the diagnosis in women patients (White et al. 2000).

It is possible that the observed gender difference in response to diagnosis is merely an artifact of the small number of men interviewed. Perhaps women and men are more similar than dissimilar and interviewing a larger sample of men would bear this out. Of course, I cannot rule out this conclusion. In the absence of more systematic data, however, I offer a few tentative and speculative thoughts concerning the intersection of gender inequality, gender ideology, and unexplainable symptoms.

Susan Greenhalgh (2001) provides a gripping account of being diagnosed with FMS (a diagnosis that she later concluded was erroneous and was eventually reversed by another physician). Her story provides an illustration of how the allure of science and the dynamics of gender combine within the clinical encounter in such a way that women patients find themselves especially vulnerable to biomedical power and authority. In her case, this resulted in her intense eagerness to please her doctor and comply with his pioneering treatment regimen that, according to Greenhalgh, resulted in an iatrogenic nightmare. None of the women interviewed in this study described an overdeveloped sense of solicitousness or an intense emotional relationship with a doctor such as chronicled by Greenhalgh. In fact, far more common was the defiant struggle to find a sympathetic doctor at all and, even then, one willing to schedule an appointment of more than fifteen minutes duration. The general point to emerge from Greenhalgh's story, however, is how the social isolation and physical and emotional vulnerability that make all chronically ill patients disposed to biomedical authority is an even greater dispositional liability for women patients. In particular, women's sense of self as more relationally defined than that of men (Chodorow 1978; Gilligan 1982), along with their secondary social status in relationship to their (primarily) male doctors, combine to make them particularly receptive to scientific authority. These factors likely heighten the salience of diagnosis for women.

Other scholars have addressed how clinical encounters between female patients and male doctors are often quintessentially gendered performances (Davis 1988; Didi-Huberman 2003; Lorber 1997; Parsons 1951). Structure dictates that each plays her or his (more or less choreographed) part in a field of power overlaid by gender, where gender inequality is effectively written into, and reproduced by, the performance (more because of unwitting complicity than conscious commitments). In summary, the role of the woman patient is *to be seen*; the role of the doctor is *to see*. Again, this dynamic heightens the salience of diagnosis for women insofar as it is the ultimate realization of this social drama.

Added to the mix is that this is a story about women whose complaints cannot *be seen*. Accordingly, as female patients seek an explanation for their medically elusive suffering, the frustrating sequence of failed medical encounters also become charged with cultural beliefs about their emotional instability, poor judgment, excitability, and tendency toward exaggeration. So it is that women with unexplainable illnesses "work hard" to be seen as a credible patient in each and every medical encounter (Werner and Malterud 2003). They do so for the benefit of their doctors but also to assure themselves. Real and perceived cultural resistance to women's authority reinforces their need for external validation. This also heightens the salience of their FMS diagnosis.

As a result of the structural and performative gender dynamic of clinical encounters between female patients and their male doctors, the pernicious marriage between subordination and self-doubt, and ideological assumptions about women's irrationality, the stakes of experiencing unexplainable illness are exceedingly high for women. Perhaps, compared with those of men, failed medical encounters more significantly erode women's sense of self and invalidate their sense of reality and, for these reasons, make the diagnostic test and the diagnosis itself far more dramatic, meaningful, and self-affirming for women. For Scott, the credentials of his diagnosing physician are bureaucratically necessary; for Laura, a name from "a man with all these credentials" is ceremonially imperative. To understand the social forces behind the FMS story, we need to understand the intense passions that motivate women to search for the biomedical validation of their suffering. The more she is denied the authority to validate her own anguish, the more she will insist it be validated in biomedical terms. Not only does this account for the dramatic quality of women's diagnostic transformations, but it might also contribute to the feminization of FMS. No doubt, men also came away troubled from medical encounters in which they are told "nothing is wrong," despite their persistent suffering. Then again, it is likely that the intersubjective demands of social reality weigh less heavily on them insofar as they are considered, and consider themselves, to be the primary authors of their own stories.

A Closing Note

As mentioned, most of the women in this study had never heard of fibromyalgia before the day they were given this diagnosis. Given the increased public visibility of FMS, however, it seems that this will be less and less the case in the future. No existing research addresses what percentage of those who suffer from FMS knew about the diagnosis or had previously self-diagnosed their conditions in advance of being formally diagnosed, nor does it provide any evidence about how these figures may be changing with time. At least in terms of the women in this study, it was not the case that those whose condition was diagnosed most recently were more likely to have heard of FMS or self-diagnosed their condition before their formal diagnosis than those diagnosed five or even ten years ago. Nevertheless, we can assume it is more and more likely that people will have heard of fibromyalgia before diagnosis and some will suspect they have the disorder well in advance of receiving an authoritative diagnosis.

This fact does not undermine the premise of this chapter. It may be the case that the diagnostic label of fibromyalgia will not come as complete news to many who suffer in the future, but that does not change many of the implications of receiving a formal diagnosis. Sufferers may suspect they have FMS, but that is not the same as having the diagnosis confirmed by a medical authority. A self-diagnosis does not bring with it the personal solace of a formal medical diagnosis. Women's FMS stories show that, before diagnosis, many fear they are dying of cancer, a fear not easily assuaged by self-diagnosis of a functional somatic disorder. In practical terms, a self-diagnosis does not bestow the cultural legitimacy or entitlements of a formal medical diagnosis, a point made at several junctures throughout the book. Lastly, the thrust of this chapter is about how women patients search for culturally coherent meaning for their illness via external authority and the profound relief that the official diagnosis of FMS presents in that endeavor. Whether they find FMS in the lay world before an official diagnosis from the medical world, is less important than that they ultimately arrive at an official diagnosis. Thus, the search for authoritative meaning and the subsequent diagnostic transformation will continue to be central to the FMS illness experience long after the diagnosis circulates as lay or commonsense knowledge.

7

Self-Help and the Making of a Fibromyalgia Syndrome Illness Identity

aving received a diagnosis marks the formal initiation of the moral career of the woman who suffers from fibromyalgia syndrome (FMS), but it is just the first step in a series of experiences that enables her to understand her illness and who she is in relationship to that illness.[1] Doctors dispense diagnoses, but sufferers quickly and eagerly seek out additional information about FMS.

> **Phyllis:** What really got me was when I started going to fibromyalgia meetings.... The doctors never explained everything, but at the meetings you learn about all this other stuff.

> **Wendy:** The doctors don't tell you anything about fibromyalgia. I left his [the doctor's] office [after being diagnosed] and I went to the library and got on the computer. I started reading stuff.... Then I realized what was going on but the doctors are no help. They diagnose you and don't tell you anything about it. They don't even tell you there are support groups.

Among the most important institutions into which the sufferer who has had her condition newly diagnosed travels, and in which she forges new affiliations, is the FMS self-help community. Eager to learn more about the illness that has long eluded her, the sufferer turns to one of the many FMS books, newsletters, Web sites, or support groups.

These self-help resources provide essential comfort for any individual learning to cope and live with chronic illness. But,

138

for FMS sufferers, who continue to face skepticism from many health care providers and other social contacts, they have a particular salience. This fact, no doubt, has significantly contributed to the dramatic growth of an FMS self-help and support community. During the last decade, several million women have joined real and virtual FMS support groups, gathered information through FMS newsletters, Web sites, and listserves, and read many popular FMS self-help books. Individuals draw on the resources of the FMS self-help and support community to manage the symptoms, but also the self-doubt and alienation that characterize the FMS illness experience. As such, self-help resources assist sufferers with their peculiar new status. They verify the formal existence of the FMS diagnosis, confirm the sufferer's FMS diagnosis, and provide tools for managing its medical marginality.

This chapter approaches FMS as a product of collective identity formation based on the experience of somatic suffering. It advances the concept of *illness identity* as a way of synthesizing the insights of two disparate theoretical bodies of literature: the illness experience literature and collective identity formation literature. In particular, using self-help books as a case in point, this chapter demonstrates how the resources of the FMS support community organize vast and dissimilar symptoms and symptom trajectories into a diagnostically bound FMS illness identity. Further, the permissive boundaries of this identity function to reduce self-doubt and alienation in a context where biomedical science is unable to make FMS visible. Whereas doctors who diagnose the condition launch the moral career of FMS patients, the self-help community facilitates the formation of an FMS illness identity.

The Concept of Illness Identity

Illness Experience

As summarized in Chapter 3, the illness experience literature describes various aspects of the lived experience of symptoms and suffering. Briefly, to restate its basic parameters, this literature provides an account of how individuals *live with* chronic illness, including how they make sense of and cope with their symptoms. It describes how individuals deflect, as much as possible, self-mortification and the erosion of the life world in the face of the restrictions that chronic illness brings and how they re-fashion a new sense of self in relationship to those restrictions. Finally, illness experience scholars look to illness *narratives*—stories of symptoms and self that construct meaning through the sequential ordering of important life events—to reveal the strategies by which individuals strive to imbue their illness with meaning and rebuild a sense of self and life world.

These deflecting and rebuilding tasks are particular arduous for sufferers who face the dual threat of debilitating, yet medically unexplainable, illnesses. Research showing how chronic pain sufferers use illness narratives to remake their life worlds is particularly helpful in delineating this process. Reflecting its grounding in cultural anthropology, this literature demonstrates how illness narratives draw on multiple sources of cultural knowledge and "local cultural orientations" (Kleinman 1988: 5). Although illness stories that individuals tell are highly personalized, they are situated "within shared cultural models" or "cultural schemas of illness" (Garro 1994: 786). For example, patients suffering from unexplainable chronic pain tell their illness stories by drawing on a cultural schema in which physical illness is recognized as "real" and psychological illness "unreal." This favors telling narratives in which symptoms are framed as physical to legitimate both the suffering and the sufferer. Likewise, in their study of chronic fatigue syndrome (CFS), Lars-Christer Hayden and Lisbeth Sacks (1998) explain how patients, drawing on a cultural template in which suffering is equated with illness, use the medical interview to narrate their diffuse suffering as *symptoms* of illness. They do so because it offers hope that the symptoms will be legitimated and, possibly, treated. Certainly, these themes are evident in FMS sufferers' narration of their symptoms and their search for a diagnosis, as described in the preceding chapters.

Although this line of investigation clearly illustrates the cultural fabric of illness narratives, it does not explore how the remaking of the self might take the form of *collective* action. More specifically, it does not address how individuals come together, using these shared cultural repertoires, in an effort to remake their individual *and collective* selves. Increasingly, the search for illness meaning has become a public and communal endeavor in which individuals make sense of their illness within self-help and mutual support communities. Patient groups now survey and interpret the cultural landscape, producing and disseminating knowledge about their own health conditions (Clarke et al. 2003).

The FMS community is just one of many well-developed, health-related support communities. The proliferation of Internet news groups, bulletin boards, listserves, and chat rooms devoted to illness make evident that, to an ever-increasing extent, people come to understand their illness by affiliating with others who share their illness. For guidance in addressing this collective dimension of the illness experience, we must turn to a second literature—that on collective identity formation.

Collective Identity Formation

In recent decades, sociologists of collective identity formation have described the social practices through which identities—shared characteristics (boundaries) that mark *us* from *them*—come to be constituted (Bourdieu 1984; Lamont 1992; Taylor and Whittier 1992).[2] Drawing on the theoretical and methodological capacities of narratives, Margaret Somers (1994: 618–619) contends that identities are constructed through "stories that social actors use to make sense of—indeed, to act in—their lives." Somers calls these stories "ontological narratives," because they are stories about who we are. Although these ontological narratives are used to make sense of an individual life, they are inherently social and interpersonal because they draw on public narratives that are attached to both small- and large-scale social networks and institutions.

People construct a sense of themselves *and* of themselves in relation to others by situating themselves in public narratives that make sense of their lives. These narratives, in turn, serve as cognitive resources that help individuals see themselves as linked to some (and distinct from others) on the basis of shared characteristics (Melucci 1988). Public narratives, thus, help individuals formulate the claims, "I am one of us," or "I am not one of them"—claims that reveal how identity exists simultaneously at the individual and the collective level. Although numerous studies have applied this framework to diverse forms and bases of collective identity formation, few scholars have explored the way in which *illness* operates as the basis for collective identity construction.

Among the notable exceptions is Carole Cain (1991), who describes how participants in Alcoholics Anonymous (AA) learn the "AA story" and, in turn, tell their own stories by locating their experiences within the archetype. According to Cain (1991:215), the AA story provides a "cultural vehicle for identity acquisition," or a narrative structure for self-meaning as an alcoholic. Similarly, Adam Rafalovich notes how collective narratives are the key to identity transformation in Narcotics Anonymous (NA). Specifically, he documents the process of "leveling," or the narrative process that homogenizes individuals and leads them to perceive themselves as "all sharing the common thread of the 'disease' of addiction" and the "identity of addict" (Rafalovich 1999: 134).

Leslie Irvine (1999) also shows how participants in codependency self-help groups, using the group's shared narrative, retell their unique personal stories to create their identity as "codependent." Codependency is not technically an illness, but it is conceptually organized within the addiction/recovery disease framework. Joan Brumberg (1992) makes a parallel claim with respect to anorexia nervosa—namely, that "symptoms" are shared via social networks and, in turn, come to form a patterned disease narrative in which identity becomes embedded. Finally, although it was not the central focus of their research, Peter Conrad and Deborah Potter (2000) mention the role of the attention deficit hyperactivity disorder (ADHD) support community and self-help books in the adoption of ADHD by an adult population.

Illness Identity

The concept of illness identity can be seen as a bridge that links the insights of the illness experience and collective identity formation literature. As established by the illness experience literature, an illness denotes the lived experience of having symptoms and suffering from them. Collective identity formation involves the understanding of one's self and affiliation with others in terms of shared characteristics (boundaries) that mark *us* from *them*. Therefore, an illness identity refers to an understanding of self and affiliation with others on the basis of shared experiences of symptoms and suffering. The theoretical and methodological use of narratives in the literature of both illness experience and identity formation directs our attention to public *illness narratives* and the investigation of how such narratives facilitate identity formation.

I will now explain how individuals work to remake their life worlds in the face of FMS by drawing on the public narratives of the FMS self-help and support community. Now that they finally have a diagnosis, sufferers can turn to these crucial public narratives to learn about their illness and affirm its "realness" in the face of its contested status. To illustrate this point, I examine the role of FMS self-help books in facilitating the creation of an FMS illness identity, or in understanding how their experience links them to others. Lest I be misunderstood, I am not saying that the fibromyalgia support community, in general, (or fibromyalgia self-help books in particular) construct FMS in the absence of "real" suffering or that individuals hysterically act out the symptoms about which they read.[3] Rather, I seek to illustrate the ways the FMS self-help and support community creates a public narrative into which individuals in distress can logically situate their symptoms to give them structure, meaning, and legitimacy.

The FMS Self-Help and Support Community

The fibromyalgia self-help and support community includes FMS sufferers and sympathizers committed to improving the quality of life for those with FMS through self-help, mutual support, education, and advocacy. Although it is clear that an extensive FMS community exists, it is not an easy task to describe its boundaries. It is a highly amorphous entity, including a handful of national advocacy and educational organizations; hundreds of disparate local support groups; a vast array of Internet sites, chat rooms, and listserves; and, an ever-expanding body of self-help literature.

Several attempts to create a national FMS umbrella organization have failed. Hence, rather than a unified national organization with state chapters and local branches, an enormous and diverse collection of local, state, and national groups exist that work to promote the well-being of FMS sufferers. One reason for the failed organizational consolidation is the varied levels of professional and biomedical orthodoxy of these diverse groups and the inability of any one group or set of groups to declare central authority over the others. The organizations staffed by, or most closely aligned with, biomedical professionals, for example, actively distance themselves from groups that might compromise their scientific credibility—a charge that becomes particularly threatening, given the already marginal medical status of the FMS diagnosis. The rapid appearance and disappearance of many real and virtual groups further inhibits community unification and standardization. The blurry line between advocacy and commerce also complicates the notion of community. One of the most popular newsletters and Web sites (Fibromyalgia Network) provides a host of customer-only resources. A glossy magazine (*Fibromyalgia AWARE*), replete with advertisements for common FMS prescriptions, nutritional supplements, and lawyers specializing in posttraumatic fibromyalgia, is published by the National Fibromyalgia Association. Nevertheless, these many distinct entities, some medically orthodox and some unconventionally "New Age"; some well established and some freshly emerging; some strictly educational and some with one foot in the commercial world, do constitute a loose community. For example, most are virtually connected to one another through a dense web or matrix of links among affiliated Internet sites.[4] The individuals, groups, organizations, and resources that are a part of this diverse matrix will henceforth be referred to as the FMS community.[5]

The amorphous and constantly changing character of the FMS community suggests the limitations of describing it in terms of its specific institutional and organizational entities. An alternative way of capturing the ethos of the FMS community is by unveiling the shared aspects of its public narratives. The core features to the narrative account of FMS, as presented in popular self-help books, posted on well-traveled Web sites, offered in popular newsletters, and articulated at real and virtual support groups, are the focus of this analysis.

Sufferers draw on the resources of the FMS community in different ways and at markedly different levels. Nearly all those diagnosed with FMS use some combination of self-help or mutual help resources generated and exchanged within the FMS community. Most sufferers have read one of the popular self-help books. More commonly, individuals read several self-help books, check their favorite FMS Web sites periodically, subscribe to one of the national FMS newsletters, and, at least occasionally, attend a local support group or enter an electronic chat room. Finally, a small number of sufferers become deeply involved in the FMS community. After reading everything about FMS that they can, they attend weekly support group meetings or become leaders of such groups, travel to regional or national conferences, and participate in one of the many national FMS organizations. To be sure, FMS sufferers vary in terms of their level of engagement with the FMS community, but few stand wholly outside of its reach in the era where mass media health resources proliferate.

Self-Help Books

A search on Worldcat (www.oclc.org/worldcat), the most extensive electronic library catalog, lists several hundred fibromyalgia self-help books. Most of these books have been published since 1996, with new books constantly coming on the market. Table 7.1 lists the five most influential books as of January 2000. The books are ranked by distribution demand, using figures from a major U.S. book distributor. Distribution ranking does not show sales per se, but shows the distribution of books into the marketplace, presumably in response to current demand. Sales figures come from publishers and they reflect the accumulated total of purchases since first publication date. In other words, distribution ranking captures the current popularity of a book, whereas sales figures capture its popularity over time.

As seen in the table, one book stands out as the most influential FMS self-help book: Devin Starlanyl and contributor Mary Ellen Copeland's *Fibromyalgia and Chronic Myofascial Pain Syndrome: A Survival Manual* (1996) (referred to henceforth as *A Survival Manual*). This book is considered by many *fibromites*—a term introduced by Starlanyl—to be the "FMS Bible." *A Survival Manual* topped the list in terms of distribution demand in January 2000, and it remains the highest ranked by demand as of January 2003. This is an impressive feat in a genre where new titles appear constantly and readers gravitate toward the newest medical information.[6] Because of its clear and persistent dominance, I organized this chapter around *A Survival Manual,* but also refer to each of the other self-help books listed in Table 7.1 as evidence in the analysis.

All the self-help books summarize the main symptoms of FMS, detail disorders that are similar to (or coexist with) FMS, outline what is currently

Table 7.1. Fibromyalgia Self-help Books in Order of Distribution Demand, January 2000 and Estimated Sales, January 2000 and January 2003

Title	Author(s)	Sales 2000 (Sales 2003)
Fibromyalgia and Chronic Myofascial Pain Syndrome: A Survival Manual	Starlanyl and Copeland	300,000 (330,000)
Reversing Fibromyalgia	Elrod	73,000 (287,000)
Fibromyalgia: A Comprehensive Approach	Williamson	87,000 (150,000)
The Fibromyalgia Help Book	Fransen and Russell	80,000 (121,000)
The Fibromyalgia Handbook	McIlwain and Bruce	*

Publisher refused to release sales figures.

known about the potential causes of FMS, and discuss current medical treatments, including alternative medicine. Each of the books is devoted to outlining techniques for managing the symptoms and the medical, personal, and workplace struggles related to FMS.

Although all five books cover the general self-help advice listed above, each promotes a particular therapeutic approach. In addition, the books differ on the basis of their authority. Some authors are medical professionals, whereas others are individuals with FMS. Devin Starlanyl is a M.D. who has FMS and myofascial pain syndrome. Finally, the books vary in their legitimacy as evaluated by the FMS biomedical research and treatment communities, although many FMS readers do not recognize these distinctions. Despite these variations, the books are remarkably similar in terms of their narrative composite of FMS, which has important implications for shaping FMS as an illness experience.

A Permissive Illness Narrative: The Symptoms and Etiology

Analysis shows that the FMS narrative presented in self-help books is highly permissive, and this permissiveness is achieved in a variety of ways. For example, perhaps the single most obvious observation regarding the FMS self-help literature is the presentation of extensive lists of symptoms that are potentially characteristic of FMS. In 1990 the American College of Rheumatology (ACR) established pain as the sole diagnostic basis for FMS. Shortly after its formal adoption, however, a committee of FMS medical experts recommended some clinical flexibility, allowing for the consideration of many additional symptoms when entertaining the suitability of an FMS diagnosis. Thus, in clinical practice, no longer are there any strictly necessary or sufficient criteria for FMS, but, rather, some degree of interpretive flexibility exists.

Self-help books take liberties with this lack of precise diagnostic criteria. All five books detail an expansive FMS symptomology. In *A Survival Manual,* the reader is asked ninety-six questions (see Table 7.2) concerning common FMS symptoms. The sheer number of possible symptoms

Table 7.2. Questions from *A Survival Manual* Concerning Common FMS and FMS/MPS Symptoms*

1. Did you have "growing pains" and chronic aches as a child? (p. 68)
2. Do you attract blackflies and mosquitoes? (p. 68)
3. Do you have bodywide achiness? (p. 68)
4. Do you have allergies? (p. 69)
5. Do you experience extreme fatigue? (p. 69)
6. Do you have mottled or blotchy skin? (p. 70)
7. Do you have loose ("double-jointed" or hypermobile) joints? (p. 70)
8. Do you crave carbohydrates or sweets? (p. 70)
9. Do you have frequent yeast infections, itchiness on the roof of your mouth when you eat tangy cheese, or bloating if you drink beer? (p. 70)
10. Do you have overgrowing connective tissue—nail ridges or beads, nails that curve under, ingrown hairs—and do you scar easily? (p. 71)
11. Do you have sleep apnea? (p. 71)
12. Do you have generalized itchiness? (p. 71)
13. Do you experience frequent frustration? (p. 72)
14. Do you experience unusual reactions to medications? (p. 72)
15. Do you have thick mucus secretions? (p. 72)
16. Do you have an inability to sweat or extreme night/morning sweats? (p. 72)
17. Do you have patches of skin with a painful network of fine veins and capillaries? (p. 72)
18. Do you have dermographia (writing with a fingernail on your skin leaves red welts)? (p. 72)
19. Do you have night-driving problems? (p. 73)
20. Do you have an extreme susceptibility to infection? (p. 73)
21. Do you have delayed reactions when you are too active physically? (p. 73)
22. Do you get the shakes? (p. 73)
23. Do you bruise easily, and do your bruises take a long while to come out and a very long time to go away? (p. 73)
24. Do you have jumpy muscles? (p. 74)
25. Do your hands feel painful in cold water? (p. 74)

Table 7.2.   *(Continued)*

26. Have you experienced a recent weight gain or loss? (p. 74)
27. Are you very sensitive to light? (p. 74)
28. Does the noise of fluorescent lights bother you? (p. 74)
29. Do some patterns (stripes, checks) make you dizzy? (p. 75)
30. Do you have electromagnetic sensitivity? (p. 75)
31. Do you experience numbness or tingling? (p. 75)
32. Have you had any serious illnesses, surgeries, or physical traumas? (p. 75)
33. Do you have motor coordination problems? (p. 76)
34. Do you experience an unusual degree of clumsiness? (p. 76)
35. Do you have sinus stuffiness? (p. 76)
36. Do you frequently have a runny nose? (p. 76)
37. Do you have trouble swallowing? (p. 77)
38. Do you have ear pain? (p. 77)
39. Do you experience ringing in the ears? (p. 78)
40. Do you have a chronic dry cough? (p. 78)
41. Do you have fluctuating blood pressure? (p. 79)
42. Do you have dry eyes, nose, and mouth? (p. 79)
43. Do you have problems with swallowing and chewing? (p. 79)
44. Do you have a prickling "electric" face? (p. 79)
45. Do you have red and/or tearing eyes? (p. 79)
46. Do you experience popping or clicking of the jaw? (p. 79)
47. Do you have itchy ears? (p. 80)
48. Do you grind and clench your teeth? (p. 80)
49. Do you have unexplained toothaches? (p. 81)
50. Do you have eye pain? (p. 81)
51. Do you have double vision, blurry vision, or changing vision? (p. 81)
52. Do you have dark specks that float in your vision? (p. 81)
53. Do words jump off the page or disappear when you stare at them? (p. 82)
54. Do you have frequent headaches? (p. 82)
55. Do you experience migraines? (p. 83)
56. Do you ever get a stiff neck? (p. 83)
57. Do you experience dizziness when you turn your head or move? (p. 84)
58. Do you ever have a sore spot on the top of your head? (p. 84)
59. Do you experience extreme discomfort when you wear heavy clothing and/or discomfort or pain mid-shoulder when you carry a purse? (p. 85)
60. Do you have pain when you write, a changing signature, and/or illegible handwriting? (p. 85)
61. Do your fingers turn color with the cold? (p. 86)
62. Do you have esophageal reflux? (p. 86)
63. Do you experience shortness of breath? (p. 87)
64. Do you have hypersensitive nipples and/or breast pain? (p. 87)

(Continued)

Table 7.2.   Questions from *A Survival Manual* Concerning Common FMS and FMS/MPS Symptoms.* *(Continued)*

65. Do you have a "frozen shoulder" (p. 87)
66. Do you have a painful, weak grasp that sometimes just lets go? (p. 87)
67. Do you have chest tightness? (p. 91)
68. Do you have a hiatal hernia? (p. 91)
69. Do you experience heart attack-like pains, rapid heartbeat, and/or a fluttery heartbeat? (p. 91)
70. Do you have mitral valve prolapse? (p. 91)
71. Do you have intestinal cramps, bloating, etc.? (p. 91)
72. Do you experience nausea? (p. 92)
73. Do you experience appendicitis-like pain? (p. 92)
74. Do you have an irritable bladder and/or bowel? (p. 92)
75. Do you have burning or foul-smelling urine? (p. 93)
76. Do you experience pain with intercourse? (p. 93)
77. Do you have menstrual problems such as severe cramping, delayed periods, irregular periods, long periods with a great deal of bleeding, late periods, missed periods, membranous low, and/or blood clots? (p. 93)
78. Do you experience impotence? (p. 93)
79. Do you have low-back pain? (p. 95)
80. Do you have sciatica? (p. 95)
81. Do you have weak ankles? (p. 96)
82. Do you get shin splints? (p. 96)
83. Do you "stumble over your own feet"? (p. 98)
84. Do you have upper/lower leg cramps? (p. 98)
85. Do you experience muscle cramps and twitches elsewhere? (p. 100)
86. Do you have buckling knee? (p. 100)
87. Do you have difficulty climbing stairs? (p. 101)
88. Do you have foot pain? (p. 102)
89. Do you have feet that are wide in front and narrow in the back, with a high arch? (p. 102)
90. Do you have tight hamstrings? (p. 102)
91. Do you experience strange sensations—numbness, hypersensitivity, "running water," "ants crawling under your skin," and so forth, on the outer thigh area? (p. 103)
92. Do you experience burning or redness on the inner thigh? (p. 103)
93. Do you have restless leg syndrome? (p. 103)
94. Do you have a staggering walk and balance problem? (p. 103)
95. Do your first steps in the morning feel as if you are walking on nails? (p. 103)
96. Do others in your family have these symptoms? (p. 104)

*From Starlanyl, Devin J., and Mary Ellen Copeland. 1996. *Fibromyalgia and Chronic Myofascial Pain Syndrome: A Survival Manual.* Oakland, CA: New Harbinger Publications.

revealed in these questions is overwhelming. For example, readers are asked if they experience body aches, fatigue, being double-jointed, allergies, abdominal bloating, difficulty driving at night, illegible handwriting, frequent headaches, shin splints, or fluctuating blood pressure. Additional questions inquire if readers bruise easily, experience frequent frustration, or crave carbohydrates or sweets.

Although the vast breadth of symptoms presented in *A Survival Manual* is unmatched by other self-help books, the other texts also present extensive FMS symptoms. For example, *A Comprehensive Approach* lists temporomandibular joint dysfunction syndrome (TMJ), sleep disorders, headaches, memory and concentration problems, dizziness, numbness and tingling, itchy and sensitive skin, fluid retention, cramps in the abdominal and pelvic area, irritable bowel syndrome (IBS) and diarrhea, premenstrual syndrome (PMS), muscle twitching, dry eyes and mouth, impaired coordination, urinary urgency, chest pain, and intermittent hearing loss (Williamson 1996: 11–13). Many of these symptoms, plus anxiety and depression, are listed in *Reversing Fibromyalgia* and *The Fibromyalgia Handbook*, and *The Fibromyalgia Help Book* adds a sense of swelling in the hands and sensitivity to the cold.

Not only are many of the FMS symptoms listed common in the general (healthy) public, threshold levels are generally not specified or are so low that almost any reader can easily match her own experience to the symptom. For example, the symptom questions in *A Survival Manual* include: "Do you ever get a stiff neck?" "Do you experience nausea?" "Do you 'stumble over your own feet'?" (Starlanyl and Copeland 1996: 83, 92, 98). In all of the popular books, the presentation of common symptoms without stated thresholds of frequency or intensity sets up a permissive illness narrative that can result in the misattribution, over-attribution, or both, of normal physical complaints as being FMS symptoms.

The books also travel on the margins of scientific orthodoxy by describing symptoms that include opposite effects, what we might call "either or symptoms." For example, among the ninety-six questions presented in *A Survival Manual,* it is noted that sometimes those with FMS do not catch any colds at all, but later on that their "immune system has no success attacking infections at all" (Starlanyl and Copeland 1996: 73). Some individuals with FMS cannot tolerate the sun, but others require regular exposure to the sun to combat their seasonal affective disorder (SAD). Some do not sweat at all, whereas others sweat excessively. Some cannot fall sleep, whereas others sleep constantly. In a variation of either or symptoms, some questions cover all possible ground, as with the following description of possible menstrual problems associated with FMS: "Do you have menstrual problems such as severe cramping, delayed periods, irregular periods, long periods with a great deal of bleeding, late periods, missed periods, membranous flow, and/or blood clots?" (Starlanyl and Copeland 1996: 93). As with the presentation of common symptoms, either/or symptoms create a permissive narrative framework for self-diagnostic confirmation.

The books also skirt along the fringe of scientific legitimacy by listing symptoms that are odd, even paranormal, fleeting, or migrating. Some of the more striking examples from *A Survival Manual* include: "Do you attract black flies and mosquitoes?" "Do you have electromagnetic sensitivity?" (Starlanyl and Copeland 1996: 68, 75). The latter point, according to the authors, accounts for otherwise unexplainable interference with the functioning of watches, computers, phones, and VCRs, as well as the enhanced ability of those with FMS to communicate with animals (Starlanyl and Copeland 1996: 75). Whereas none of the remaining popular books describes paranormal symptoms, they do claim that FMS symptoms can appear and then disappear, or appear and then quickly and unpredictably reappear elsewhere on the body. In sum, the books promote the notion that FMS symptoms can change or migrate on a day-to-day or sometimes hour-to-hour basis.

The self-help literature, thus, creates a highly permissive composite of FMS by presenting a vast list of common symptoms, offering no (or unclear) thresholds for the number or severity of symptoms, and detailing symptoms and symptom characteristics that fall outside, or on the margins of, scientific orthodoxy. Each of these aspects is captured in the following passage from *A Comprehensive Approach*:

> It is important to remember that having one or even a few of these symptoms does not necessarily mean that the diagnosis is fibromyalgia. But if you have low back pain and x-rays show no problem with your spine, and you have what appears to be a bladder infection and the tests come out negative, and you have aches and pains that come and go in various, unpredictable parts of your body—in fact, if you have any combination of symptoms described in this chapter, fibromyalgia may be the cause of your problem (Williamson 1996: 13).

The books also create tremendous narrative flexibility through their description of the likely *causes* of FMS. In the absence of biomedical consensus, the self-help books can be fairly unrestrained in presenting etiological possibilities. This includes describing many possible causal mechanisms that have never been clinically tested and others that have received no empirical support, despite substantial inquiry. *A Survival Manual* mentions heredity, sleep abnormalities, "triggering events" (including physical and emotional trauma), behavioral factors, biochemical (including hormonal) changes, immune dysregulation, and environmental disturbances as some of the many possible factors contributing to FMS. Williamson (1996) lists metabolic dysfunction, immune disorder, heredity, illness or injury, and prolonged stress as possible causes. Harris McIlwain and Debra Bruce (1996) mention a cycle of disturbed sleep, reduced physical activity, depression, and pain, as well as menopause, aging, serotonin deficiency, and postviral effects.

As explained in the books, any number of factors can cause FMS, but the actual relationship between these factors and the onset of FMS is vague and indeterminate. The result is a highly confused description of FMS onset as seen in the following quote from *A Survival Manual*:

> In FMS, a triggering event often activates biochemical changes, causing a cascade of symptoms. For example, unremitting grief of six months or longer can trigger FMS. It's sort of like "Survivors Syndrome." Cumulative trauma, protracted labor in pregnancy, open-heart surgery, even inguinal hernia repair have all been triggering events for FMS. Life stressors can overwhelm the body's balancing act, turning life itself into an endurance contest. Note, however, that only about 20 percent of FMS cases have a known triggering event that initiates the first obvious *flare* (Starlanyl and Copeland 1996: 13–14).

Similarly, from *Reversing Fibromyalgia*:

> [C]lose to 100 percent of the fibromyalgia victims I have personally worked with have all experienced a long period of undue stress or emotional trauma—whether it be an automobile accident, divorce, a long illness, growing up in a dysfunctional family, experiencing abuse as a child, or some other type of trauma. It is reported that these triggering events probably do not cause fibromyalgia, but rather they awaken or provoke an underlying physiological abnormality that is already existent (Elrod 1997: 16).

This horoscope technique of hooking the reader by attributing life-changing significance to widely shared aspects of human experience is present even in the most medically orthodox of the books, Jenny Fransen and I. J. Russell's *The Fibromyalgia Help Book*. This book outlines several contending causal explanations, including muscle abnormalities, physical and emotional trauma, depression, stress, and neurotransmitter abnormalities, all the while being careful not to overstep existing medical evidence. Nevertheless, in their cautious effort to describe several tentative etiological theories, they set the conceptual table with many speculative possibilities from which the reader can pick and choose in framing her own FMS illness narrative.

In sum, readers learn that the disorder can be triggered by multiple factors, either internal or external to the individual; it may not have a trigger at all; and weeks, months, or even years can separate "triggers" from symptom onset. Consequently, a specific etiologic agent, risk factor, or disease onset is not required to confirm the existence of FMS. Together with the flexibility in symptomology, the lack of a clear causal framework creates a highly permissive FMS illness narrative.

Invisibility and Illness Affirmation

Each of the self-help books speaks to the invisible nature of FMS. More specifically, each recounts the distress associated with experiencing symptoms that are indiscernible to both medical and lay observers. The following remarks from *A Survival Manual,* for example, describe how the invisibility of FMS results in the unmaking of the life world.

> As an FMS patient, you have probably been burdened with a long history of undiagnosed illness. Because your condition is more or less invisible, friends and family many not believe you when you say you hurt, so you may also be suffering from a loss of self-esteem. In other words, you may be deprived of the normal support network that forms around a chronically ill person because 'you look just fine.' And without the support of family and friends, you may well withdraw from others to conserve what little self-esteem and energy you have left (Starlanyl and Copeland 1996: 14).

Similarly, from *The Fibromyalgia Help Book:*

> One of the most frustrating aspects of fibromyalgia is that others cannot see or feel the magnitude of the pain you are experiencing. Family or friends may remark about how well you look. This is distressingly inconsistent with how terrible you feel. . . . Thus, fibromyalgia can be described as an invisible, ongoing nightmare that others cannot see or feel. Being trapped in this nightmare may cause you to doubt your own sanity, which may contribute to depression and lead to withdrawal from society into lonely isolation (Fransen and Russell 1996: 5).

Addressing the gap between the lack of objective biomedical indictors of FMS and the subjective experiences of those with FMS is a principal goal of the self-help literature. Readers are assured that they are not crazy and that FMS is real. Self-help books repeatedly cite two interrelated points to affirm the reality of FMS: (1) the symptoms of FMS are real because others share them; and (2) these shared symptoms are the basis of an established and recognized medical diagnosis.

In the face of social invalidation and isolation, solidarity around shared symptoms verifies the existence of FMS and, therefore, serve as an important resource for remaking the sufferer's life world. This is clearly evident in the following passage from *A Comprehensive Approach.*

Most importantly, you will know that you are not alone, and that the discomfort you experience is *not* 'all in your head.' . . . People with fibromyalgia feel better, mentally and physically, when they can share information and support. . . . Hearing from others with similar experiences validates you as a human being and improves your self-esteem (Williamson 1996: 4–5).

In the self-help literature, the existence of the FMS community is an affirmation of the sufferer and the sufferer is an affirmation of the FMS community. *A Survival Manual* offers a language for the sense of community among those with FMS: "I coined the word 'FMily' to describe the special bond those of us who have fibromyalgia all share. We often have more in common with our fellow fibromites . . . than we do with members of our family" (Starlanyl and Copeland 1996: 8).

The existence of the diagnosis, readers are told, also affirms the reality of their FMS experience. The adoption of FMS by established medical authorities is summarized in defense: "The American College of Rheumatology, American Medical Association, World Health Organization, and the National Institutes of Health have all accepted FMS as a legitimate clinical entity. There is no excuse for doctors 'not believing' in its reality. It's real" (Starlanyl and Copeland 1996: 13). Moreover, readers are warned not to misunderstand that the *syndrome* designation does not make fibromyalgia any less legitimate than a disease. *A Survival Manual* explains:

> *Diseases* have known causes and well-understood mechanisms for producing symptoms. FMS is called a *syndrome*, which means it is a specific set of signs and symptoms that occur together. FMS is called a syndrome. . . . Don't let this categorization fool you into thinking that fibromyalgia is any less serious or potentially disabling than a "disease." Rheumatoid arthritis, lupus, and other serious afflictions are also classified as syndromes (Starlanyl and Copeland 1996: 9).

McIlwan and Bruce (1996: 9) simply dispense with the syndrome or disease distinction altogether and, instead, use the terms interchangeably in summarizing the disorder's prevalence: "Even though this has been a commonly misdiagnosed and misunderstood syndrome, fibromyalgia is the most common arthritis-related disease next to osteoarthritis."

Accordingly, readers are encouraged to get a new doctor if theirs blames them for their symptoms or treats them as though their symptoms or FMS do not really exist. For example, the following is from *A Comprehensive Approach*:

> If your doctor responds to your symptoms by acting as though you are an impossible complainer, or telling you that your problems are all in your mind, or saying that if you will only learn to control stress (or lose weight, or both) your pain will disappear, you may need a different doctor (Williamson 1996: 17–18).

Williamson goes on to give concrete tips for finding a doctor who believes in the authenticity of FMS. Likewise, *A Survival Manual* provides a worksheet for interviewing doctors to assure that they are "fibro-friendly," that is, that they believe FMS is a legitimate medical condition and are sympathetic to FMS sufferers (Starlanyl and Copeland 1996: 356–357).

The books also reinforce the credibility of the diagnosis by telling readers about the many sufferers who persevered and finally had their condition diagnosed by providers who knew about the existence of FMS and its diagnostic criteria. For example, the self-help literature is peppered with accounts of the struggle toward, and relief on receiving, an FMS diagnosis. The following account from *A Survival Manual* is typical.

> It isn't unusual for those who are fibromyalgia patients to feel a profound sense of relief when they learn they have a recognized illness and they come to understand that it isn't progressive.
>
> If this has been your experience, you may cry with relief at not having to doubt yourself any longer. At last, someone believes you and believes in you. You really do have these symptoms, and you are no longer fighting the world alone. Debilitating self-doubt can be replaced with appropriate self-care (Starlanyl and Copeland 1996: 8).

That so many people had exactly the same experience of being demeaned and ignored by doctor after doctor, only to be vindicated in the end, powerfully adds to a discourse of authenticity. The shared catharsis of such a powerful diagnostic experience corroborates the validity of FMS.

The Subjective Salience of the FMS Narrative

The overall salience of the FMS narrative is that it finally provides the sufferer with a framework for talking about her embodied experience that is in line with her subjective sense of it. Rather than a bundle of confusing and meaningless symptoms scattered across time, the FMS narrative provides a coherent and orderly chronicle to a series of unfortunate events. The following passage from *A Comprehensive Approach* captures this point well.

> Fibromyalgia was the reason for my constant muscle aches and joint pains, and for the stabbing pains that from time to time made me catch my breath to keep from crying out. I found that the crampy diarrhea I had when I was younger was probably caused by fibromyalgia. I learned that fibromyalgia was the reason I could swell up like a balloon, gaining as much as five pounds of water weight overnight, usually losing it within a day or two. My poor coordination; the knee that sometime forgot to catch my weight, landing me in heap on the ground; the bursitis-like pain that a doctor

once told me was all in my head; the sciatica that put me in bed for three months when walking became impossibly painful, although my doctor at the time could see no reason for the pain—these things and many more are associated with fibromyalgia.

I concluded that I had had fibromyalgia since childhood. As a little girl, I was teased to the point of despair by schoolmates, teachers, and family for my clumsiness and poor coordination. When I told my mother about my aches she merely replied that pain was a normal part of living and that I should stop complaining. My adulthood was no better. . . . Doctors labeled me a hypochondriac and offered tranquilizers, sleeping pills, and psychiatric referrals (Williamson 1996: 2–3).

Fibromyalgia syndrome creates a framework for making sense of extreme pain, but, as revealed in the above passage, it also bends to incorporate the more mundane frustrations of everyday life, including clumsiness and water weight gain. The following discussion of "fibrofog" from *A Survival Manual* also captures the capacity of the FMS narrative to frame ordinary annoyances as symptoms.

Perhaps you psych yourself up to go the grocery store and arrive only to discover you've forgotten your wallet. You return home, retrieve the wallet, and set out again. After you reach the store you realize you've left your shopping list and coupons at home. . . .

Steam irons get stored in the refrigerator. Freshly made milk drinks go on a shelf, where they silently turn into a dismal green mold. You transpose letters when you write and you do the same with figures when you are trying to balance your checkbook (Starlanyl and Copeland 1996: 171).

The unbound nature of the FMS narrative allows the individual to situate "symptoms" across his or her life course, ranging from the profound to the trivial, as both major events and everyday hassles are folded into a coherent story: a childhood marked by severe injury and abuse as well as the normal feelings of youthful awkwardness; an adulthood of great physical and emotional distress as well as forgetting needed items at the grocery store or neglecting a dirty cup. The FMS narrative, therefore, offers a way of "remaking" the world by creating an overarching framework that gives order and meaning to past, present, and future symptomology (broadly defined). In the sociological sense, the diagnostic narrative of FMS, drawing many of its specific elements from the self-help community, functions as a narrative of selfhood.

Specific and Unique: The FMS Narrative Paradox

The most fascinating aspect of the FMS narrative presented in the self-help books is the tension between two potentially contradictory claims. On the one hand, readers are assured that FMS is a *specific* condition, as stated unequivocally in *A Survival Manual*: "It is important to understand that FMS is not a catchall, 'wastebasket' diagnosis. 'FMS is a specific, chronic non-degenerative, non-progressive, noninflammatory, truly systemic pain condition—a true syndrome' " (Starlanyl and Copeland 1996: 9). On the other hand, each person's FMS is *unique* in terms of onset, intensity, duration, and symptoms. For example, from *A Comprehensive Approach:* "The important thing to remember as you read the discussion of signs and symptoms is that no two people experience fibromyalgia in exactly the same way" (Williamson 1996: 8). A few pages later, Williamson evokes the legendary blind men and the elephant: "Fibromyalgia is a lot like that elephant. Each of us who has FM experiences it slightly differently, depending on which symptoms we find most distressing. . . . Each of us has a part of the truth, but none of us sees the whole disorder" (1996: 10). Whereas Williamson tells readers they may have fibromyalgia if they have *any* combination of symptoms described in her book, the authors of *A Survival Manual* advise readers that even their ninety-six questions "by no means [capture] all of the possible symptoms associated with FMS" (Starlanyl and Copeland 1996: 104).

The self-help literature presents FMS as a vast collection of ubiquitous and vague symptoms not restricted to a specific beginning (etiology or onset), intensity (severity), or trajectory (symptom course). Nearly any combination, order, and intensity of symptoms (even normal "symptoms" or symptoms not presented in the text) can be situated within the FMS narrative. Beyond the ACR criteria, which are both controversial and imprecisely applied, no specific standards exist by which an individual's symptoms or symptom course would disaffirm FMS. Within the self-help literature, the reader finds an unbound narrative that offers many points of entry, tremendous flexibility, and few thresholds of exclusion. The permissive or unbound narrative, therefore, creates flexibility to account for the uniqueness of an individual life, a unique narrative of selfhood.

Nevertheless, all the variability between individuals is effectively rendered conceptually superfluous by collapsing it under the unified diagnosis of FMS.

> Forty-one-year-old Janis told of hurting everywhere on her body; even sitting in a straight-back chair brought tears to her eyes. Sarah, a young mother of two, felt throbbing pain all over her body as well as disturbances in deep-level, restful sleep, accompanied by sadness or depression. Mike felt a piercing pain in his neck and shoulder, accompanied by sluggishness, that came on suddenly after a car accident. While these patients had different manifestations of pain and fatigue, the symptoms were all the result of fibromyalgia (McIlwain and Bruce 1996: 8).

Consequently even as the FMS narrative is a permissive narrative of self-hood, it is simultaneously a homogenizing narrative that facilitates collective identity formation. Dissimilar experiences are tied together through the FMS diagnosis, which, in turn, allows individuals to embrace a common identity as fibromyalgic or "fibromite." The self-help literature, as a public narrative, facilitates the construction of a distinctly *collective* FMS illness identity that links an individual to others through a constellation of overlapping symptoms and channels them into a new subjectivity focused on their illness and its management.

The Interviews: Reading FMS Self-Help Books

Having summarized key aspects of the FMS narrative presented in self-help books, the question arises of how individuals read these texts. What impact, if any, do these books have on an individual's illness experience? The remainder of this chapter addresses this question.[7]

The women interviewed in this study differ in their level of engagement with self-help literature. Only Phyllis said she never read any FMS self-help books. Nevertheless, she does read the educational handouts provided by her support group leader, which summarize popular and medical FMS publications. Emily reported having read several books early in her illness but found them depressing, discouraging, and of little use. In contrast, the most common response to questions concerning FMS self-help books was: "I've read almost everything on the market" (Sally); "I've read just about everything out there" (Wendy); "I read everything I can get my hands on" (Alice); and "I've probably read them all" (Evelyn). Indeed, most of the women have read many self-help books. Several took them off shelves and coffee tables while being interviewed and their preferences tend to confirm the figures in Table 7.1. In line with national sales figures, by far the most commonly mentioned book was *A Survival Manual* or as Margaret put it: "I did read the one, the purple book that *everyone* reads." It is understood that she means *A Survival Manual.*

Even as all but one of the women has read FMS self-help books, they evaluate their importance differently. Paula prefers to read the peer-reviewed FMS medical literature and regrets that most self-help books, with the exception of *The Fibromyalgia Help Book*, contain what she considers to be misinformation. Courtney and Meredith report having read several books, but they no longer recall any specific details, lapses they both attribute to their "fibrofog," a term introduced in *A Survival Manual.* Most women, however, describe being positively and deeply affected by the FMS self-help books and focus on the importance of *A Survival Manual* in particular. As a group, the women draw on this book (and others) to organize and give meaning to their own symptoms and to affirm the "realness" of their subjective experience in the face of biomedical uncertainty.

Primarily, the women are amazed at how well the details in *A Survival Manual* fit their own experiences. To many, the book represents being understood. Its pages give witness to the very nature of their experience. Laura concisely captures this common feeling: "Well, parts of the book honestly read as if someone was following me around with a movie camera." Others describe the common process of reading through the book, page by page, and finding their symptoms.

> **Wendy:** It was funny. When I first got the book, I took a highlighter and marked the things that I had, and after three pages the whole thing was marked. I'm a classic case!

> **Ellen:** There was a lot of stuff in there that I could identify about myself. Like, oh yes! I have this, and I have that, this symptom, and that problem, and so forth.

Two women, Joan and Morgan, read from *A Survival Manual* during the interview, turning to specific pages and explaining how peculiar it was when they first saw their own symptoms flawlessly described.

> **Joan:** Just thumbing through the book while we are talking...pages 95 through 122...I have something just like it or similar. Parts of each question I can pick up on....I can see myself in different parts of the book.

> **Morgan:** Ordinarily I can't read long...but I kept reading because it was freaky how she wrote about everything I have. Right here, [she starts reading from page 73 of the book] I can't drive at night because I have bad night vision. I get every cold that comes along. When I overdo, it always takes a few days for my muscles to really, really ache. When I get hungry, I get shaky hands. I bruise easily. I hate fluorescent lights and I did not understand why. And I starred this one [she reads directly from page 75 of the book]: "I must also make sure that I don't look at escalator steps. They are ridged, and the lines and movement are enough to drop me in my tracks." I still remember reading this and thinking, "My God, she has exactly what I have!"

From the extensive list provided in *A Survival Manual,* readers identify their specific symptoms. The permissive narrative allows them to select those symptoms that are most salient, without excluding themselves for failing to display the vastness of the symptom composite. In large measure, this has to do with the widespread understanding that no two people express FMS the same way.

Sally: We don't have the same symptoms. Everyone is different, but we have stuff in common. The book [*A Survival Manual*] explains that.

Wendy: I am not saying we all have the same symptoms, or even the same symptoms in the same order and that is what is so frustrating to the doctors. You need to find a doctor who will put all your medical history together like Devin [Starlanyl] does in this book.

The women find their many symptoms captured on page after page of *A Survival Manual.* More significantly, the FMS narrative provides them with tools to organize and make sense of their seemingly unrelated, unexplained, and distressing symptoms. These symptoms are all apart of a coherent whole—FMS.

Rachel: For me the image of connect-the-dots comes to mind. She has taken all of these symptoms that you can look at as little dots and she ties them altogether with me at the center. . . . Dry eyes, irritable bowel syndrome, and irritable bladder syndrome. She has taken all of these symptoms and made sense of them.

Cindy: For such a long time you think you're crazy because you have all these crazy symptoms. When you start reading about how they are all pieces of FMS, you finally see the whole . . . it finally makes sense.

Wendy: TMJ, the pain, the concentration, the memory, vision, irritable bowel, irritable bladder, it [*A Survival Manual*] goes on and on and on. Dermatitis, athletes' foot . . . it all connects right back to fibromyalgia. . . . It's stuff that none of us realized was part of it . . . they are all a part of FMS.

Readers are encouraged to be mindful of the vast number of complaints attributable to FMS, or the "stuff that none of us realized was part of it." Following are powerful examples of how this dynamic unfolds.

Doris: I was reading about it one night, about how black flies are attracted to the skin. . . . I was sitting on the couch and I just started crying because I have had that problem for ten years probably. When there are flies in an area they'll always land on me . . . it just bowled me over. I mean, what a weird thing. . . . I couldn't believe it when I read it after having that problem for so many years.

Morgan: I never knew why I hated fluorescent lights or why striped shirts and escalators made me dizzy. I knew that I had all these things but I didn't know they were all apart of the same thing.

The FMS narrative allows the reader tremendous flexibility to organize "symptoms" within its boundaries and, thus, increases the likelihood of framing normal physical complaints as FMS symptoms. For instance, Joan notes how *A Survival Manual* allows her to challenge someone who doubts the importance of her seemingly common symptoms: "When someone says, 'It is just a bruise,' you can say, 'No' in your own words by using the book, because the book *is* your own words."

Drawing on the self-help books, readers learn that other routine annoyances are actually symptomatic of FMS. Sally mentions tripping; Laura brings up spilling food; Cindy cites blotchy skin and poor handwriting; Christina refers to transposing numbers. Each of these is listed as FMS symptoms in *A Survival Manual*.[8] Likewise, sufferers frequently attribute symptoms normally associated with aging to their FMS. For example, having recently reread *A Survival Manual,* Joyce remarks:

> **Joyce:** I had totally forgotten about fibrofog. I just thought I was having a succession of "senior moments,"... but actually there is a reason for this.

Based on their reading of self-help books, others also respecify normal aging as symptomatic of FMS.

> **Wendy:** Your eyes—everyone says it's just because you're over forty, but that's not it. My vision has changed drastically.... She [Starlanyl] goes into all of that in the book.

> **Jessica:** There are a lot of symptoms that you think are just because you're getting old but they're not. I mean...I ache, I forget things, my vision is lousy, and if I sneeze and don't cross my legs I pee my pants. But you learn that these are part of fibromyalgia, not just about getting old.

The women have years of inexplicable symptoms for which to account. Recall, on average, they experienced six and half years of acute symptoms before having their condition diagnosed and an average of nearly fourteen years separated the onset of their first symptoms and their diagnosis.[9] This reality, read onto the highly ambiguous causal framework presented in the self-help books, facilitates the organization of symptoms and experiences into an extensive life-narrative. Many of the women retrospectively see the thread of FMS throughout their lives.

> **Phyllis:** I mean, now that I read things about it, I think this started when I was real little, *real* little.

> **Valerie:** Now that I understand fibromyalgia, I think I've probably had it since high school.

The latitude set up by the self-help books allows individuals to frame years of somatic distress as possible causes for, and outcomes of, their FMS. The following comments, made in reference to *A Survival Manual,* illustrate the potential of the FMS narrative to retrospectively give meaning to years of distress.

> **Ellen:** It's *me* in that book. My life is that book. It told me so much about myself. I was flabbergasted. . . . I witnessed a traumatic event when I was only ten months old. They say I suffer from PTSD [posttraumatic stress disorder] because of this. I don't remember because I was a baby, but I was subconsciously affected. . . . In seventh and eighth grade I was having a lot of accidents and breaking bones. By the time I was seventeen . . . it really intensified. . . . I had lots of injuries, two abusive relationships, had some other traumatic things happen, deaths in the family, so it could've been aggravated by any of that. Then I got real sick. I was sick from December until the end of March with flu and a sinus infection. Exactly four years later, three days after my car accident, the same thing happened. . . . I went through the same thing. I was sick for three months. . . . I went through all these long illnesses and it was because of my FMS.

In their study of those who suffer from multiple chemical sensitivity (MCS), Kroll-Smith and Floyd (1997: 11) found that individuals struggle to create a "practical epistemology" or a way of making sense of their "obscure bodies" in the context of professional biomedicine's confusion about the disorder. Despite the lack of scientific support for MCS, as a cognitive framework it is logically consistent with the distress sufferers experience. In a similar fashion, the FMS narrative offers a practical, subjectively logical, account of somatic distress. The following is a particularly telling example of how an extensive history of distress is practically framed through the FMS narrative.

> **Maude:** I think I had this when I was a kid. I was abused. I remember telling my mother that I ached and hurt. I did a whole series of paintings when I was a kid about having no arms and legs because I couldn't get comfortable at night. My mother used to say, "It's growing pains, you're neurotic, I am going to send you to a psychiatrist.". . . Then I had that back injury and I've been in pain ever since. . . . I've been on the verge of suicide, of wanting to kill myself but not wanting to die. . . . I've been in pain for years . . . and now I know what it is. . . . The fact there's a book out there validates the things I've been going through for years.

The FMS public narrative provides a practical and logical account of readers' broadly felt distress but, as seen in Maude's comments, it also has an important validating quality. Seeing their experiences described and explained on the pages of a book is tremendously important to nearly all of those interviewed, especially after enduring a long period where no one understood or believed their experiences. The self-help books not only make readers finally feel understood by someone else (indeed an entire community), but they also provide a framework of self-understanding after a long period of self-doubt. The women read *A Survival Manual* and other self-help books as self-validating and as evidence of the reality of FMS.

> **Laura:** There were some chapters that would reduce me to tears . . . because this is exactly what my life is like. That helped from the standpoint that this has not been my imagination.

> **Christina:** It validated that there was something out there. Other people knew what you were going through. . . . There were so many things going on with me that I started to think that maybe I am a hypochondriac. When I read the book it helped me understand that I am not crazy, I am not imagining this. It is real. It made me feel better to know that it is real and not all just in my head.

As seen in Christina's comment, an important link undoubtedly exists between self-validation, community, and the "realness" of FMS. Others echo the affirmation and hope represented by a community of fellow sufferers.

> **Morgan:** You read someone explain your own symptoms like you wrote it yourself, but once you realize you have the exact same thing that others have, you breathe a sigh of relief. I know that sounds bad because you don't want anyone else to be so sick but you know what I mean.

> **Hannah:** I do think that the reading has helped me just in terms of my own psychological ability to cope with this because it offers validation that this is real and that you're not nuts and that there are other people that are dealing with it and coping with it.

The diagnostic solidarity of symptoms and sufferers forms the basis of an FMS illness identity. Readers come to understand that they are linked to others symptomatically, and this link validates the symptoms and self. Or, as Wendy says of *A Survival Manual*;

> **Wendy:** I think I speak for all of us when I say . . . it made everything that we have real! Devin's book, and some of the other fibromyalgia books, have brought us all together.

Conclusion

The search for illness coherence and selfhood are part of the experience of any serious or prolonged illness. Increasingly, the nature of this search has become collective as individual sufferers turn to self-help resources and communities that have grown up around myriad chronic illnesses. This is most dramatically seen with the proliferation of Internet news groups, bulletin boards, listserves, and chat rooms devoted to illness. In addition to this general cultural trend, particular features of the FMS experience (or the experience of any contested illness) make both the search for meaning and the collective nature of that search even more profound.

The focus of this chapter has been on the role of self-help books in shaping the FMS illness experience, but the narrative presented in these books is similar to that of other resources produced and exchanged throughout the FMS community. FMS Web sites, real and virtual support groups, and organizational newsletters all advance a similarly permissive and homogenizing narrative. In books, at groups, or on the Internet, individuals read their unique personal experiences from and onto the FMS narrative and, in the process, give meaning to a wide range of individual suffering. At the same time, the narrative diagnostically links individual sufferers to others, thereby leveling variance among them and forging a sense of commonality. Sufferers' sense of shared experience encourages the formation of an "FMily," as represented here in an image from a popular FMS Web site (Figure 7.1). The FMS public narrative, thus, represents a cognitive resource through which individual experience is validated and endowed with meaning and an illness identity is established.

Benefits of FMS illness affiliation exist, as do the benefits of self-help participation for anyone struggling with chronic illness. Finding their experiences described on a book page or computer screen signifies to sufferers that they are being understood by others and offers them a forum for self-understanding amidst the "biographical disruptions" of illness

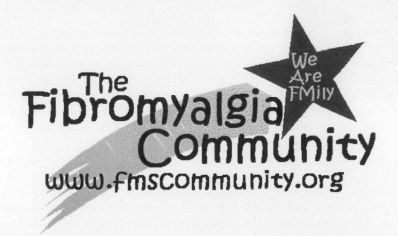

Figure 7.1   "We Are FMily." Used by permission of The Fibromyalgia Community.

(Bury 1982). Moreover, illness affiliation provides crucial fellowship, support, and encouragement through the sharing of personal struggles and victories. Practical advice for managing symptoms and the daily personal and workplace tensions related to symptoms can also be acquired. Finally, affiliation can result in political power and subsequent democratic claims on public resources. The FMS support community has made each of these benefits a reality for FMS sufferers. In addition to the benefits of restored self-hood and fellowship, as captured in women's comments presented in this chapter, political gains have also been made. In 1999, for example, FMS sufferers became legally eligible for federal disability compensation—in no small part, because of the lobbying efforts of the patient advocacy organization Fibromyalgia Network.[10] Even though it remains difficult for sufferers to be awarded disability compensation solely on the basis of the FMS diagnosis (actual figures are unknown), this is a clear symbolic victory in that it recognizes that individuals with disabling symptoms should be entitled, as citizens, to these public resources.

Nevertheless, there are also less positive or more troubling consequences of FMS illness affiliation and identities. Several points warrant our focused consideration. Illness identities channel individuals into new subjectivities intensely focused on their illness and its management. Everyday frustrations, normal aging changes, minor infirmities; years of complex distress, trauma, and abuse; and serious but common conditions are all presented as "symptomatic" of FMS. Sufferers perceive more and more of everyday life as part of their FMS, not because they are gullible or mentally unstable, but because FMS is a compelling cognitive category that can accommodate a great number of distressing experiences within its narrative structure. At the same time, subsuming such a wide range of unpleasant experiences within a disease model risks both denying the inherent suffering of the human condition (thereby weakening our ability to confront its inevitability) and failing to search for *nonmedical* reasons for particular forms of women's distress. In short, by medicalizing such a broad assortment of human suffering, FMS runs the risk of either anesthetizing or depoliticizing women's everyday lives. Although having their condition diagnosed does not appear to have obvious negative consequences on women's well-being, neither does medical management result in tangible improvement in their symptoms or levels of functional disability.

Finally, consider the role that illness identities play in the ongoing social construction of FMS. Whatever FMS may or may not be in biomedical terms, the widespread adoption of FMS as an illness identity is a social fact that cannot be denied. Because the FMS narrative is such a compelling and encompassing cognitive framework, it has the capacity to lend coherence and meaning to a wide variety of perceptions and sensations, confirming their existence as "symptoms" of FMS. Even as biomedical science is unable to make FMS visible, sufferers' interaction within the FMS community constructs a powerful sense of common experience through which the existence of FMS, as a discrete and unitary entity, is affirmed. Through social interaction, biomedical heterogeneity comes to acquire meaning as experiential homogeneity.

Ties That Bind and the
Problem That Had No Name

Social and behavioral scientists, including many feminists, have criticized biomedicine for its inattention to social variables and their role in health and illness. The dearth of social information with respect to fibromyalgia syndrome (FMS) is typical in this respect. Published clinical research commonly gives consideration to the sex, race, and age of those with FMS, but makes little use of this information beyond describing sample parameters and matching patients and controls along these dimensions to check for "spurious" influences. Moreover, as in biomedical research in general, these variables are conceptualized as solely biological, without consideration of their cultural dimension. Community prevalence studies, which reveal how common FMS symptoms in the general public are, tend to be more attentive to a broader range of social characteristics (e.g., level of education, occupation), but such studies are rare. What is more, as part of the general biomedical enterprise, community prevalence studies also tend to approach variables such as sex and race primarily as biological characteristics.

I have already addressed how these features of biomedicine's orientation contribute to the "present absence" of gender from FMS research. Not only is FMS a feminized disorder, but the particular ways in which it is feminized offer important insights into its character and point to the limitations of the existing FMS debate. This chapter provides an analysis of the available social epidemiology of FMS in an effort to bring the central claims of this book into sharper focus—namely,

166

that FMS is both a socially constructed category of biomedical knowledge and a cognitive structure that gives meaning to women's distress.

Social Epidemiology of FMS

Sex and FMS

The prevalence of FMS by sex has already been addressed. To summarize, clinical and community studies differ in their estimates of the female-to-male ratio of FMS sufferers. As we might expect, given women's higher rates of health care utilization, clinical studies reveal the disorder to be even more dramatically feminized than community prevalence studies. Among those clinically diagnosed with FMS, women overwhelmingly predominate; even among nonpatient populations, however, it is estimated that between 75 and 90 percent of those who meet the FMS criteria are women (Hawley and Wolfe 2000; White et al. 1999a).

Race and FMS

Racial and ethnic minorities, especially African Americans, are significantly underrepresented among those identified with FMS in both clinical and community prevalence studies. In many clinical studies, there is no mention of race (Yunus et al. 1989); in others, all the patients are identified as white (Yunus et al. 1981); and, in still others, racial and ethnic minorities account for a small percent of the total patient sample (Wolfe et al. 1990). A recent clinical study exploring the presence of FMS among patients with lupus concluded that being white is positively associated with FMS and being African American is negatively associated with FMS (Friedman et al. 2003). Community level data on the racial and ethnic composition of those who meet the FMS criteria are limited. The most recent and extensive community level study, for example, fails to mention the racial or ethnic composition of the FMS population at all (White et al. 1999b).

Nevertheless, there are some relevant community prevalence data on the race and ethnicity of FMS sufferers. For instance, a study conducted in a city were whites made up 80 percent of the population found that 90 percent of those identified as having FMS were white (Wolfe et al. 1985). In other words, whites were overrepresented among those with FMS. Other studies provide interesting, albeit fragmentary, details about race and FMS. For example, one community study found that FMS does not occur among Pima Native Americans (Jacobsson et al. 1996). Another community study examined 162 low-income minorities who reported musculoskeletal pain and self-perceived arthritis (Bill-Harvey et al. 1989). The group was 80 percent women, two-thirds African American, and one-third Hispanic. The subjects were given a rheumatological examination and 42 percent of Hispanics met the criteria for FMS, compared with only 3 percent of African Americans. Because this study was limited to subjects who already reported significant musculoskeletal pain, these rates are significantly higher than would be found in the general minority population. In relative terms, however, the study clearly shows that FMS is extremely rare among African Americans compared with Hispanics.

According to the best available evidence, it is estimated that well over 90 percent of those within the general public who meet the American College of Rheumatology (ACR) criteria for FMS are non-Hispanic whites (Hawley and Wolfe 2000; Wolfe et al. 1990). By comparison, roughly 69 percent of the total U.S. population is non-Hispanic whites, indicating that this group is significantly overrepresented among those with FMS (U.S. Census Bureau 2003). Even Hispanics, the most prevalent minority among those with FMS, are significantly underrepresented in relation to their share of the total population. Perhaps as many as 5 percent of those who meet the FMS diagnostic criteria are Hispanics of any race, a category representing 12.5 percent of the total U.S. population.

Class and FMS

The distribution of FMS along class lines in the United States has not been directly investigated. This is in keeping with the general tendency in the United States to deny or downplay class as a potentially important variable in a wide range of social and natural scientific research. Consequently, with the exception of one recent study, what we know about the relationship between class and FMS comes from studies conducted outside the United States. The one U.S. study found that nearly 40 percent of patients with FMS had incomes less than 1.85 times the established poverty level, compared with 21 percent of patients without FMS (Wolfe and Michaud 2004:695).[1] A community prevalence study conducted in London, Ontario, found that a lower household income increased the odds of having FMS (White et al. 1999: 1570). In a unique community prevalence study conducted in Finland, 3,434 subjects who screened positive for musculoskeletal disorders were given physical examinations (Makela and Heliovaara 1991). Even among this group with existing musculoskeletal disorders, FMS was relatively uncommon: only fifty-four cases—less than 1 percent of the sample. Interestingly, of the 1,596 white-collar professionals in this study, not one met the diagnostic criteria for FMS. Fibromyalgia was essentially absent among affluent urban residents and more common among urban poor and rural residents.

A Swedish study also found a relationship between FMS and occupational rank (Hallberg and Carlsson 1998). This study was based on interviews with twenty-two Swedish women with fibromyalgia. Among other things, the researchers found that unsatisfying work—including that which was low status, strenuous, and tedious, and that over which women exercised little control—characterized the occupational settings of women with FMS. With few exceptions, these women had low levels of education and worked in female-dominated occupational categories in the "reproductive" sector, including health care, childcare, and eldercare services.

America's aversion to the notion of persistent class inequality and the corresponding ideological alliance with meritocracy result in the use of education as a proxy for class in social and medical research alike. Of course, education is strongly correlated with class, but the economic and occupational benefits of education differ by class background (as well as by race and gender).[2] But, given the dearth of U.S. data on the link between class and FMS, exploring the relationship between education and FMS is worthwhile.

Overall, there is strong evidence that education is inversely related to FMS symptomology in both clinical and community populations. A large community prevalence study conducted in Wichita, Kansas clearly demonstrates this relationship (Wolfe et al. 1995). For example, this study found that the odds of not completing high school were three and a half times higher among those who met the FMS criteria than among those who did not. Clinical studies also reveal the negative association between the prevalence and severity of FMS symptoms and educational attainment, including a reduced likelihood of completing high school and of graduating from college (Goldenberg et al. 1995; Wolfe and Michaud 2004).

Data from outside the United States, including the Canadian and Finnish studies noted above, offer a similar picture. Kevin White et al. (1999) found that patients with FMS were less likely than other pain sufferers to have completed high school and less likely than the general public to have a college degree. Makela and Heliovaara (1991) found a dramatically higher incidence of FMS among those who attended only primary school compared with those who graduated from high school. In another study, intended to explore ethnic differences among Israeli immigrant women diagnosed with FMS, researchers found that Sephardic patients had more frequent and more severe symptoms than did Ashkenazic patients, but the observed differences were primarily the result of *educational* not ethnic differences (Neumann and Buskila 1998). In sum, the negative relationship between FMS and education is found in community and clinical populations both within and outside of the United States.

Together, these data on income, occupation, and education, suggest that FMS is associated with *less* rather than more class privilege. These findings are somewhat unexpected, given the prevailing assumptions about the upper middle-class nature of women's somaticism. Chronic fatigue syndrome (CFS), for example, is sometimes snidely called "yuppie flu" as a way of denoting its association with persons from privileged class backgrounds with the time, so to speak, for indulging sickness. At the same time, however, there is a curious underrepresentation of women from certain social groups that are associated with the very least class privilege, namely, racial and ethnic minority women. Startling, for example, is the fact that among low-income African Americans (most of them women) with musculoskeletal pain, only 3 percent met the FMS criteria (Bill-Harvey et al. 1989).

Summary of Race and Class Differences

Building on the available social epidemiological data, we can conclude that FMS is primarily found in women, but disproportionately so among non-Hispanic, white women. Additionally, a well-established negative relationship is seen between education and FMS. Evidence also points to an inverse relationship between FMS and occupational rank, including a link to service sector labor characterized by low status, low wages, and low levels of workplace autonomy. Therefore, FMS is not primarily a disorder that affects privileged women, but neither is it found uniformly across all categories of disadvantaged women. Community prevalence studies that are not biased by differences in health care access or utilization consistently find racial and ethnic minorities underrepresented among those who meet the FMS criteria.

It is worth pausing to make a key clarification. It is important not to reify these figures themselves as evidence of some underlying *essence* of what is, after all, a socially constructed category. These figures tell us what social characteristics are empirically related to the presence or absence of FMS criteria. Therefore, all that we actually know from these social epidemiological data is that women are more likely than men to subjectively confirm the presence of the ACR criteria and that white women of modest means are more likely to subjectively confirm the presence of the ACR criteria than are more affluent white women or women of color.

With this caution in mind, the social epidemiology of FMS sits awkwardly within the parameters of the existing FMS debate. It is hard to imagine, for example, how an account of FMS as a neurobiological disorder resulting in centralized sensory misperception could account for the distinctive gender, class, and racial composition of those who meet the FMS criteria. The conceptual gap between the model's assumptions and the social epidemiological data seems insurmountable. Framing FMS as an affective spectrum disorder characterized, in full or in part, as the misperception of common stresses on the part of a psychologically disturbed individual also cannot address the distinctive social characteristics of those who meet the criteria. The neurobiological, as well as the psychogenic and behavioral accounts, frame FMS within the constraints of the biomedical model. In particular, FMS is *endogenously* conceptualized, or conceptualized as a disorder caused by factors *inside* the individual. Yet, the social epidemiology points to *exogenous* or social and cultural factors not reducible to individual biological or psychological characteristics. Even FMS research that attempts to focus on "psychosocial" factors is restricted from a genuine investigation of sociocultural influences because of its conformity to the clinical mode of investigation that severs individuals from the social world in which their symptoms emerge, are perceived, and then endowed with meaning.

I have argued that the FMS diagnosis (and the debate surrounding it) is only the most recent of a century-long series of largely unsuccessful efforts to make sense of women's complex somaticism using the orientation and tools of biomedicine. I have also argued that FMS functions as a cognitive category that gives meaning to women's broadly felt distress. How then might we proceed to advance our understanding of the suffering that characterizes FMS in light of these claims and the social epidemiological data presented above? The answer: principally by locating women's FMS stories in the social worlds in which their symptoms originate and gain meaning.

We are aided in this task by the fact that the women in this study compare closely with the social epidemiological parameters described above. All of the thirty women are white, one is Hispanic. Of the twenty-six women who participated in the in-depth interviews, four graduated from a four-year college, nineteen graduated from high school, and three never completed high school or its equivalency. Although more than half of the women are currently not working, as a group their work histories can be summarized as performing low-wage, feminized jobs in the clerical and service sectors. For example, with the exception of one registered nurse and one elementary school teacher, none of the women spent her work life in a professional occupation as defined by the Department of Labor. Eleven of the women work or worked in clerical occupations (e.g., secretary, cashier, bookkeeper), three as technical health care workers (e.g., licensed practical nurse, nurse's assistant), eight as other service sector workers (e.g., hair stylist, fast food worker, housekeeper), one as a manual laborer, and one reported never having worked outside the home. In line with the social epidemiological studies summarized above, the women in this study are primarily white, working- or lower middle-class, mostly with little education beyond a high school diploma.

We can say, with no judgment implied, that those who suffer from FMS are "unremarkable"; they are typical American white women. Women's FMS stories, therefore, are stories about women's well-being, more generally, and illustrative of the complexities of their worlds of pain.

FMS, Worlds of Pain, and the Ties That Bind

Meredith and Betsy

In the early 1960s, Meredith left high school before graduating, married Jack, and started a family. She and Jack have been married for nearly forty years and their three children are now grown. They raised their family and still live in a town where the main industry has suffered decades of economic contraction. Jack is a manual laborer for the town's atrophying industrial employer. Meredith never formally worked outside the home but, in addition to being a full-time homemaker, she worked informally cleaning houses to make extra money. Now that she is no longer able to do such physically demanding work, it is clear she and Jack are barely making it financially. They own a small and modest home and, although it is well cared for and warmly decorated, as with other homes in the neighborhood it reflects the hard times of a community marked by sharp economic downturn.

Meredith is fifty-five years of age, although she looks considerably older and more frail than her age would suggest. Her body movements are especially slow and deliberate; she moves in apparent pain. A rheumatologist told her that an injury she received at age thirteen is likely responsible for her fibromyalgia. She recalls the event that broke her pelvis.

> **Meredith:** I just stumbled. I was running to school and I was running late and I fell on the railroad tracks and I got up really quickly because I didn't want nobody to notice that I fell. So I just brushed my dress off and off I went to school. When I got to school they told me that I had hurt my back really bad and said that my parents should take me to the hospital. But at that time my parents said they couldn't afford it, they just didn't have the money. And so I just learned to cope with it.

She did learn to cope with it for many years and it was not until she became pregnant in her early twenties that her FMS really developed.

> **Meredith:** It was when I started having children.... Well, it seemed like with each of my children my back got worse.... It seemed like when I was carrying the baby the lower part of me started in hurting so much. It hurt in the front and then in my lower hip. There was an awful lot of pressure on my hip. So then with each child it got worse.

During her third pregnancy she developed complications and nearly died during delivery. It was a great disappointment to Meredith that she was unable to become pregnant again. But, even without further pregnancies, Meredith's pain persisted and her condition deteriorated. Now, however, she had to care for three children. In addition to constant, shooting pains running down her arms and legs, Meredith developed a host of additional symptoms that troubled her and for which she sought medical attention. Then, twenty years ago, after living with acute symptoms for more than ten years, Meredith had her condition diagnosed as fibrositis, the diagnostic precursor to fibromyalgia, by a pioneering FMS clinician researcher.

Meredith's diagnosis was established ten years before the ACR criteria were formally adopted, but her symptoms have shown little or no improvement during the twenty years she has been treated for FMS. Not only have Meredith's symptoms failed to improve but, as she ages, they have also become less manageable. Her current FMS symptoms include severe pain in her back, hips, knees, arms, and hands, as well as migraine headaches, extreme fatigue, sleeping difficulties, irritable bowel syndrome (IBS), depression, and throat and eye irritation. Even with minimal exertion, Meredith becomes exhausted; her legs swell and her pain becomes intense. She has to lie down several times each day to minimize her symptoms, but even then she is never without pain and fatigue.

Meredith's primary care physician oversees her treatment for FMS, which consists exclusively of pharmaceuticals. She takes an alarming number of daily medications, including some to combat side effects of those she takes for her primary symptoms. She takes several different pain medications, multiple antidepressants, a few prescriptions to help her sleep, and others to control her stomach upset. Added to the mix is hormone replacement therapy; Meredith had a complete hysterectomy many years ago when she was diagnosed with endometriosis and fibroid tumors. She is concerned and frustrated about the large number of medications she takes and their seeming lack of efficacy. She jokes about being a "drug addict" as she sorts through a basket containing dozens of pill bottles.

> **Meredith:** I don't even use them all. I just feel that if I find, you know, that they're not going to do any good then there ain't no sense in using them. I get so disappointed with it sometimes because you feel like your taking all these things and they're not helping.

Despite her prescription arsenal, Meredith remains in constant pain and is unable to work or keep up with her household chores. She also stopped helping at the local hospital where she had long volunteered. Indeed, by any definition Meredith is disabled, although she has never applied for any disability compensation. In one breath, Meredith describes her disabling symptoms while she anxiously talks about her need to find a job to help make ends meet. The financial pressures on Meredith and Jack have become acute lately. Recently, Jack was ill and unable to work for several months and, although he is back at work now, they were forced to use up their modest savings during his convalescence. "It's hard," Meredith notes, "when it gets down to the bottom." Maybe, she continues, she could learn some computer skills and find a job that would not be as physically difficult as her old cleaning jobs. On some level, however, Meredith seems to understand the improbability of a woman fifty-five years of age without a high school diploma getting a computer job in a town and a nation in the midst of economic recession.

Meredith and Jack have always had a traditional division of labor; he has been the breadwinner and she has assumed responsibilities for the domestic sphere. Not only has this division, in part, resulted in their current precarious financial situation, but Meredith also feels the pressures it creates in terms of Jack's response to her illness.

> **Meredith:** I wish he would help out more. . . . I don't think he really understands it at all. I think that he thinks that it's all in my head. It seems like that if there's things to be done around here he can't see what needs to be done and sometimes I will ask him to do it but if he's watching TV he'll say "wait a minute." I don't like that. . . . I've always done everything for him, and he's never had to wash a load of clothes in his life or anything like that. I just feel that he should be good to me in return and help me out when I need it, but he doesn't.

The entrenched nature of their traditional division of labor is made apparent when Jack returns home during the middle of the interview. Meredith had just finished explaining the extreme pain she is currently experiencing in her legs, arms, and hands, and her desire for Jack to help out more in the home. Yet, when Jack enters the kitchen, she quickly busies herself waiting on him, handing him a glass of soda and ice. Jack did not ask for a soda. Meredith did not ask if it was wanted. Despite the lack of words, their mutual expectations perpetuate a domestic situation that is ripe with painful contradictions. Meredith herself spoke directly of these contradictions when, at the close of our interview, I asked her if she had any questions for me.

> **Meredith:** Do you think that stress has a lot to do with this [FMS]? Because I am under a lot of pressure and stress with my husband all of the time. . . and I think a lot of my sickness has been caused to happen because of the stress. He gives me really low self-esteem.

But, it would be misleading to end Meredith's narrative with her lament regarding Jack. Overall, she is warm, giving, and upbeat. She does not think of herself as a victim, nor does she feel tremendous pity for herself. Instead, she balances her personal sadness and frustration about her illness against her thankfulness and hopefulness.

> **Meredith:** I think, well, I've got to think of it this way: there are worse things. There's other people who have worse things that happened to them ... so I have to thank the Lord that it's not to where I'm incapacitated. . . . I just hope some angel will come down someday. I've tried to help out so many other people, I have. And now I think it's time that the Lord would start giving me a little bit of that back [she laughs]. I am very glad for my family though.

Although Meredith seems emotionally able to manage the limitations her illness places on her own life, she begins crying when she talks about her youngest child, her daughter Betsy who was diagnosed with FMS three years ago. As Meredith and Betsy sit side by side it is easy to see the closeness mother and daughter share and the sympathy and compassion they feel for one another.

> **Meredith:** It's a horrible thing that my daughter inherited it from me. . . . I feel terrible. . . . When I found out she had to get this stuff, oh, it just broke my heart. I just thought, "It's not fair."

Betsy cannot remember the last time she slept particularly well and, yet, even in her state of visible fatigue she reveals a wonderfully tenacious spirit. She is currently in her late twenties, works part time as a secretary, and is married to Steve, a frequently unemployed construction worker. Betsy recalls a sickly childhood.

> **Betsy:** I was always sick as a child. I always had a cold or the flu and didn't feel well at all. The doctors did all kinds of tests on me to try to figure out what it was but then nothing would show up. It was so frustrating to me, because I felt sick, I felt ill, and they just basically kept saying that there was nothing wrong with me.

When Betsy started menstruating, her periods were irregular and painful. Her family physician put her on birth controls pills to treat her menstrual symptoms when she was thirteen. Although this regulated her periods, Betsy still felt badly all the time and doctors remained unable to find anything wrong with her general health. This state of affairs— mundane but frequent sickness—went on throughout her teenage years.

After graduating from high school Betsy found a job as a secretary, but her persistently poor health made working difficult. Sitting for long periods was especially painful and Betsy took frequent sick days and cycled from one job to another. Then, her already poor health and spotty work history worsened when she broke both elbows in an accident when she was twenty-one. Betsy simply never recovered. The accident left her in intense pain and, when her pain and fatigue persisted month after month, Betsy started drinking heavily in an effort to escape.

It was around this time that Betsy and Steve married. The newlyweds started off under the cloud of Betsy's pain and excessive drinking. After yet another injury, she spent most of her time on the couch in pain, drinking and sinking further into blackness. She tried every type of pain medication, moving up to ever-stronger narcotics. Eventually, she was taking several Percocet tablets every few hours and drinking heavily, but her pain and despair only intensified. Around this time, her physician prescribed an antidepressant, but Betsy was convinced that depression was the *result*, not the cause, of her problem. She knew there was a real answer. One day, after reading her mother's FMS educational materials, she realized that she, too, had fibromyalgia.

> **Betsy:** I noticed that it was all the same symptoms I complain about when I go to the doctor's office. Before all this I had said [to the doctor] "What about fibromyalgia?" and he said, "No, no, you're way too young, it can't be that, it has to be something else." So then I went through those papers and I highlighted every single symptom that I had in there. It was practically everything.

So Betsy made another appointment with her primary care physician and convinced him to refer her to a rheumatologist who confirmed her suspicions. Like her mother, she has fibromyalgia.

Betsy is greatly relieved to finally know what she has, but the doctors have had little to offer her. She now takes morphine and it has reduced her pain considerably. The morphine has a number of unpleasant side effects, but she views them as a necessary evil: "My only choice is to take morphine or die." With the pain at least partially under control, Betsy is more functional now than she was a year ago and she has even returned to a part-time job. In addition to morphine and antidepressants, she takes a host of medications, including muscle relaxants and sleeping pills. When she feels well enough, Betsy attends Alcoholic Anonymous (AA) meetings, which she also sees as an important part of her treatment. The most effective therapies for Betsy have been various methods to calm and relax her. Bath salts, massage therapy, and biofeedback bring her some degree of calm; they help her find what she calls "a quiet happy place with nothing going on."

Betsy acknowledges that a strained marriage runs parallel to her illness, thereby giving context to her search for a "quiet and happy place." Describing Steve's impatience with her prolonged illness, she becomes visibly upset.

Betsy: Oh, he was awful! He was the worst, worst, worst husband in the world! He was so verbally abusive, so degrading,... he was terrible. "You should be walking by now.... You're just lazy;. You're a piece of shit." He used to call me some really, really bad names and he was just very verbally abusive. If I was laying there he would come and rip the covers off of me and yell, "Get up! Get up and do something! Come on, you need to be active! You're just being lazy!"

For a period of years, both Betsy and Steve were drinking steadily and, combined with the pressures of Betsy's health, their relationship grew even more highly charged.

Betsy: For a while we were in a really bad place where he would just keep on me and keep on me and I would get so angry and I would say, "Steve, you have to stop or I am going to lash out. I'm going to hit you. You've got me really worked up." This would be after a couple of drinks.... This one night I threw a pillow at him as hard as I could. I picked up the phone and I called an 800 number for help and I talked to like fifteen different people before I got to someone who could finally help me.

The conflict only made her illness worse and, out of desperation, Betsy told Steve she planned to leave him. In response to the threat, Steve became more sympathetic and, so far, Betsy has decided to stay with him. Nevertheless, she seems realistic about the likelihood that he will become abusive again.

Betsy: I hope he stays in a good place now. I hope he doesn't go back, but if he does I'm totally prepared to leave him, because I can't handle it. It's too hard on me.... It makes me really depressed and tends to make me more suicidal. I just can't live that way.

Meredith responds to her daughter's assertiveness and bravery:

Meredith: I'm so proud of what she's done with him. I tell her, you know, "Don't ever go through what your mother did."

In both Meredith and Betsy's cases, the pain of FMS seems overdetermined. Indeed, there are few mysteries about their general ill health at all. Their symptoms emerge in the context of both serious physical injuries and the struggles and conflicts of everyday life. Physical pain and the pain of martial conflict, a deficit of support, lack of opportunity, financial dependence, and economic want become indistinguishably intertwined.

When Meredith's parents could not afford the necessary medical care for her broken pelvic bone, she learned to endure the pain while her teenage body slowly and partially healed. The childhood injury made each of her pregnancies a major physical sacrifice. As a poorly educated woman married to a working-class man in lean economic times, her strategies of endurance and sacrifice have been drawn on again and again over time. Years of caring for her husband, often by denying her own physical and emotional suffering, has not resulted in the accumulation of care-giving capital that Meredith can cash in on her own behalf. This denies her crucial support in the face of her own illness and the gross inequity produces intense personal anguish. Now, with many constrained decisions behind her, she has few options available and looks out at the physical, financial, and marital road ahead with anxiety and a heavy heart. Meredith embodies the burdens of too much scarcity and sacrifice and too few resources and sources of support.

Betsy did inherit many of the more painful aspects of Meredith's life. She is more fortunate in that she graduated from high school and her work history, even if sketchy, gives her the confidence and resources to live independently, if necessary. It is also significant that she remains childless; Meredith had her three children by age twenty-six. These material differences give Betsy more options and fewer constraints to respond to marital discord. Yet, even these differences do not fully transcend the similarities between mother and daughter. Among other things, Betsy inherited the persistence of class and gender inequality, as they come together in the form of restricted options and inadequate resources. With limited education and low-status work experiences, her opportunities are only a modest improvement over her mother's, but perhaps they will give her enough leverage to make demands on her husband for an equitable and supportive relationship.

Gender, Class, and the Intergenerational Continuity of FMS

Meredith and Betsy's lives exemplify the complexities of women's suffering and highlight the difficulties of capturing those complexities in terms of a biomedical model. At the same time, however, their experiences correspond to an extensive body of scholarship that demonstrates how women's typical domestic and work lives can contribute to their ill health. This scholarship, discussed in Chapter 2, elucidates how gender inequality in the workplace and domestic context can directly or indirectly undermine women's health by exposing them to physical, economic, and emotional hardships. The types of work women typically do (e.g., care-giving and emotional work at home and in the workplace, low-status jobs in which they are subordinate to authority, repetitive motion tasks) can all negatively impact women's well-being. Moreover, their concentration in low-wage work frequently results in their economic dependence on male partners and can limit their abilities to create equitable and compassionate relationships.

Of course, not all women have low-status and low-wage jobs (nor do all men work in high-status and high-wage positions). Some women, like their privileged male counterparts, have more resources to respond to crises and to control and adjust their everyday situations in ways that protect their health and well-being. For example, because male-dominated occupations are more likely to receive paid vacations, as well as paid sick and disability leave, than occupations that are feminized, women who hold historically male jobs also receive these benefits. This discrepancy furthers the health disparity between women and men, as well as between more and less privileged women (Rieker and Bird 2000). At the same time, for those with inadequate personal resources and support, access to health care can become one of the few avenues available for securing some remedy. As Judith Lober (1997: 65) observed of working-class women in the late nineteenth century, receiving "medical attention" might well have been "better than no attention." This observation is all the more relevant in the early twenty-first century when most working-class women are covered under some form of health insurance, however precarious and eroding that coverage may be.

Meredith and Betsy's FMS experiences are easily situated in the context of these arguments regarding women's health. Moreover, although their experiences are unique, the overdetermined quality of their FMS is something that is found in the accounts provided by most of the women in this study. Nevertheless, these women are genuinely *puzzled* about their lack of physical well-being. Recall Alice, whose FMS experience opened this book. She experienced a car accident, caring for her dying mother, the grief of her mother's death, and an ineffective surgery. Yet, rather than interpreting her ill health as the cumulative effects of these experiences, she remarks, "There was just no explanation for it." Similarly, Valerie describes how her general frailty and pain intensified into troubling illnesses over time.

> **Valerie:** With each tragedy in my life, the pain was more severe. Childbirth, I had two very difficult pregnancies and deliveries. I never seem to recover as fast as most people. So if I would have a simple infection it would take longer to recover.... Then things progressed. I had a death of a spouse, moved to a new area, and once again trauma, massive trauma, just one right after another.... The pain never went away and it got so severe. I didn't know what was wrong with me.

Evelyn, too, became ill in a complicated web of distress. Following a divorce (about which she avoids offering any details), she became a single mother of two teenaged children trying to make ends meet by working fifteen-hour days as a temporary worker. She became run down and vulnerable to persistent infections that simply would not go away. Eventually, she literally collapsed in response to losing her job.

> **Evelyn:** Then, like on my last day of work I just sort of fell down to the ground and I didn't want to live anymore. They took me to the hospital, and I stayed there for three days.

Yet, Evelyn is genuinely puzzled by her pain and fatigue and, together with her doctors, tries to make medical sense of them.

Other women in this study tell of the succession of painful physical, economic, and emotional experiences and events that led to their FMS. After her divorce, Cindy was so broke she had to borrow money from her parents to pay her rent and so she begrudgingly started taking on double shifts in her job at the local nursing home. But then, she injured her back lifting a patient at work and, after two failed back surgeries, at fifty-five years of age, Cindy has now moved in with her brother, his wife, and their four children.

After years of widowhood, Doris remarried, but her second marriage was brief and painful. The marriage was bad from the beginning and, in quick succession, Doris had an ulcer, a persistent stomach infection, two serious work injuries, back surgery, and was forced to leave her job. "There was no rhyme or reason to it," Doris reflects back on her illness onset.

Jessica dropped out of high school. When she was twenty-three years of age, she had three children under the age of four and an ex-husband who offered her no financial assistance. She began experiencing a never-ending series of colds and infections but her health worsened with the tragic death of her young son. Puzzled by her constant pain, she went from doctor to doctor in search of a medical explanation, eventually being diagnosed with FMS.

Finally, Phyllis's symptoms first became pronounced during a period of sustained physical abuse from her husband. She could hardly breathe, her heart raced constantly, her muscles ached with tension, and she was unable to sleep. Yet, somehow, she reflects on these symptoms by saying, "There was just no reason for it."

Other such stories abound—some more, some less remarkable—but the point need not be dramatized further. FMS represents a constellation of physical and emotional hardships and distresses in the absence of mobilizable resources or meaningful explanations. In other words, the hardships of women's lives combine to form an enveloping matrix of distress that can be meaningfully organized as FMS, even as the biomedical particulars of their experience are markedly different.

One of the most interesting ways this is seen, and the reason for focusing on Meredith and Betsy, is the intergenerational continuity of FMS.

Biomedical research recognizes the common familial occurrence of FMS; although some researchers speculate that FMS has a genetic component, no evidence yet corroborates such a conjecture (Buskila et al. 1996; Yunus 1998). In addition to Meredith and Betsy, another mother and daughter pair are among those interviewed and fully half of the remaining women in the study mention that they have at least one female relative with FMS. In some of these cases, women's relatives have had their conditions diagnosed as FMS. In most cases, however, women diagnose their own relatives (both living and deceased) based on their experiential knowledge of FMS. Whether a hereditary association is ever determined, what is clear from these family ties is how the FMS narrative gives meaning to the intergenerational persistence of women's distress. As Meredith put it, "It's a horrible thing that my daughter inherited it from me. . . . It's not fair."

Insofar as FMS makes sense of women's own painful lives, it can also be applied outwardly to make sense of the similarly painful lives of women relatives. Following are just a few comments from women reflecting on the parallels between their own worlds of pain and those of their mothers, sisters, and daughters.

> **Wendy:** I know for a fact my mother had fibromyalgia. She was never diagnosed with it. She had twenty-five surgeries. I have had sixteen. . . . My daughters—I can see the stuff in them that I had at their age. The yeast infections, the bladder problems, the chronic cystitis, the headaches. Katie was in an accident about two years ago. She has been a mess ever since. Of course, they don't appreciate hearing this; . . . it means that they have this. Especially at her age—she was only nineteen—and the only thing she has to look forward to is being like her mother. Tammy is twenty-three and if something dramatic happened to her like an accident she would end up just like me. As I'm sitting here I'll tell you my mother had this. I think both my sisters have it and both of them are in big denial. One of them is a nurse and every time she lifts a patient and hurts her back she is out of work for three years. But she will not admit that she has FMS.

> **Courtney:** So during that time as well, when I had finally realized that that's what it was, . . . the symptoms were really prominent in the sister that is older than I and one that's just younger than I. They had both suffered way longer than I had, and I told them to get tested and since then they have both been diagnosed with fibromyalgia.

> **Hannah:** I know my sister is beginning to feel like she has the same thing and she's been going to a rheumatologist. More and more I've heard that it might run in families.

Our culture promotes the dual ideologies of individualism and meritocracy. Our society, we are told, is one in which life's rewards and riches are distributed based on our individual efforts and achievements. With-out denying the importance of individual agency, such ideas thwart our ability to see the ways our personal crises are often attributable to social forces well beyond our individual control. Such ideas undermine our ability to develop what C. Wright Mills (1959) called a "sociological imag-ination," a type of self-consciousness in which one is able to make sense of personal troubles in the context of larger social and historical factors. In a society that undermines the development of such an awareness, FMS functions as one of the few available explanations for the everyday *and* dramatic suffering that marks many women's lives, including that which persists across generations of women. In a culture that cannot see how personal *troubles* might be public *issues* (Mills 1959), heredity stands in for entrenched inequality. Stated briefly, women's descriptions of the persis-tence of FMS across generations of female relatives give meaning to larger forces of social reproduction.

Sick and Tired of Being Sick and Tired

Fibromyalgia syndrome has been described as the end point of a con-tinuum of distress-related symptoms (Hawley and Wolfe 2000). This po-sition appears consistent with the argument presented above regarding the overdetermined nature of FMS symptoms and of women's health, more generally. Accepting this interpretation, we are still left with one seemingly incongruous fact that begs for an explanation: why is it that certain women, who are subject to some of the most persistent and pro-nounced stresses and hardships, nevertheless are *underrepresented* among those whose condition is diagnosed as FMS? In the U.S. context, this is most obviously the case with respect to racial and ethnic minorities—especially African Americans. Black women in the United States are es-pecially unlikely to meet the FMS criteria. This is true, although they do have high rates of other stress-related disorders (e.g., heart disease, ul-cers, hypertension) (White 1990: 11).

African American women tend to inhabit a variety of different sub-cultures within the larger black community and these differences have variable health consequences. Nevertheless, persistent health disparities exist between black and white women (Franke 1997). Compared with white women, black women (and certain other racial and ethnic minority women) "have higher rates of reproductive problems, higher rates of mor-bidity, and higher rates of mortality from most causes and in virtually ev-ery age group" (Wingard 1997: 43). Not only are age-adjusted death rates for black women significantly higher than for their white counterparts, so too are rates of chronic morbidity and disability (Geronimus 2001;

National Center for Health Statistics 2000). The distinctive stresses that characterize many black women's lives manifest themselves in their over-representation with respect to a host of stress-related conditions. For instance, compared with white women, "hypertension in black women is characterized by higher incidence, earlier onset, longer duration, higher prevalence, and higher rates of hypertension-related mortality and mor-bidity" (Gillum 1996: 385). In fact, "rates of hypertension-related mor-tality for black women [in the United States] remain among the highest in the industrialized nations" (Gillum 1996: 385). Likewise, the mortal-ity gap between black and white women from cardiovascular disease is 65 percent in the United States (Franke 1997).

Despite this otherwise bleak picture, black women are significantly un-derrepresented, not only among those with FMS, but also among those suffering from a host of stress-related, functional somatic syndromes that primarily affect women. African American women are less likely to have headache disorders than white women (Hamelsky et al. 2000), and are sig-nificantly underrepresented among those with interstitial cystitis (Parsons et al. 2000). The racial composition of temporomandibular joint (TMJ) dysfunction sufferers has not been extensively studied, but existing re-search suggests that the disorder is significantly less common among black than among white women (LeResche and Drangsholt 2000). The racial and ethnic composition of those with multiple chemical sensitiv-ity (MCS) is also not fully known, but, like FMS, most of the clinical- and community-based samples have been largely non-Hispanic, white women (Baldwin et al. 2000).[3] Black women's underrepresentation among those suffering from these highly feminized stress-associated disorders, given their poor physical health and their high levels of economic, occupa-tional, and social distress, presents a puzzle.

The Cultural Meaning of Pain

Certainly, one possible explanation that needs to be considered is the fact that white women, on average, have greater access to health care and, therefore, greater access to functional somatic diagnoses. This could be part of the reason for some of the patterns noted above. In the case of FMS, however, the underrepresentation of black women is found not only in the clinical context but also in community prevalence studies that are not biased by racial differences in access to health care. This suggests that unequal access to health care alone cannot explain the low numbers of black women who meet the criteria for FMS. Instead, I propose that we search for the solution to this puzzle in terms of cultural dispositions toward chronic distress and the institution of medicine and how these dispositions differ between black and white women.

In the 1950s and 1960s, Mark Zborowski (1969) studied ethnic differences in pain expression among male hospital patients. To the modern reader, Zborowski's conclusions capture discomforting stereotypes. For example, he found that "Yankees" were withdrawn and stoic in the face of pain, whereas Jews and Italians were more expressive and animated with their pain complaints and wanted not to be left alone in their suffering. Despite our contemporary unease with these stereotypes, Zborowkski's research opened the way for thinking about how cultural context and meanings shape the experience of pain (Good et al. 1992). From this perspective, contemporary anthropologists have explored more systemically how history and local cultural worlds shape the experience and meaning of pain (Good et al. 1992; Ware and Kleinman 1992). For example, Arthur Kleinman (1988: 23) argues that the current "epidemic" of chronic pain in North America has a particular historical and cultural meaning.

> The epidemic of chronic pain complaints in North America suggests that pain has peculiar present-day significance. . . . Perhaps North American culture's ideology of personal freedom and the pursuit of happiness has come to mean for many guaranteed freedom from the suffering of pain. This meaning clashes strikingly with the expectation in much of the nonindustrialized world that pain is an expectable component of living and must be endured in silence.

The notion that normal life is free of pain and suffering is a relatively recent cultural disposition (Morris 1991). Such a shift in disposition is partly the result of secularization, which has distanced us from religious world views in which suffering is understood as central to the human experience. Processes of medicalization also reinforce our expectations that no level of suffering is acceptable (Illich 1976; Markens 1996). In effect, we have become so susceptible to viewing pain and suffering as *abnormal* and so impatient with the experience of pain that we seek quick solutions to ensure our freedom from its grip (Illich 1976; Morris 1991).

Take the example of menstrual distress. Premenstrual syndrome (PMS) is a constellation of physical and mood distresses unheard of in much of the world and among members of some ethnic groups in the United States, but it is increasingly commonplace among white, especially middle-class, North American women. Indeed, an entire industry has been created around the alleged disorder (Markens 1996). Many non-Westerners regard PMS as yet another example of the unwillingness of Westerners to endure any pain and suffering, no matter how limited and predictable (Kleinman 1988: 24).

Nevertheless, the dominant cultural assumption concerning the abnormality and avoidability of suffering may not be equally shared across all social groups. Rather, both history and social stratification determine the possibility of framing freedom from suffering as the norm.

Black Women and the Cultural Routinization of Pain

The birth of "second wave" feminism is commonly associated with the publication of Betty Friedan's *The Feminine Mystique* (1963), in which she recounts the emptiness experienced by the mid twentieth-century suburban housewife. Even while the suburban housewife seemingly had everything she was supposed to want—a providing husband, children, a home, and material comfort—she remained curiously dissatisfied, a dissatisfaction Friedan called "the problem that has no name." Black feminist scholars were among the first to point out the limitations of Friedan's account and its lack of applicability to the lives of women who neither had it all nor were at a loss for an explanation for their dissatisfaction (hooks 1984). Put simply, black women did not need Friedan's consciousness raising movement to become aware of their dissatisfaction or its social causes.

As a result of the persistence of gender, race, and class inequality, contemporary black women remain unlikely to experience their distress and compromised well-being as a "problem that has no name." More than ten years ago, the National Black Women's Health Project and *The Black Women's Health Book* (White 1990) brought this perspective to the fore. In a collection of essays, Angela Davis reflects on the forces that impact black women's well-being. "While our health is undeniably assaulted by natural forces frequently beyond our control, all too often the enemies of our physical and emotional well-being are social and political" (A. Davis 1990: 19). However, as noted by Opal Palmer Adisa (1990: 11–14), black women are not without resources for dealing with the hardship and suffering of their lives.

Since then [forced slavery], all African American women have been seeking a rocking chair and the sun light to rock themselves well.

All African American women may not have rocking chairs, but we have each other. The best doctor, best medicine, best antidote for what ails us is the mirror reflection of ourselves: our friendships, our bonds, the comfort we seek and the support we receive from each other. . . . We use each other's strength and tenacity to fight the stress that would put us in our graves before our time.

. . . [W]e have learned to create balm-yards to mix potions and perform a laying on of hands, to share our magic so that we can vanquish the stress that slaps us in the face everyday. . . . We rock while we talk about needing a new job that pays better and provides benefits, about being taken for granted....

It's because stress is hemmed into our dresses, pressed into our hair, mixed in our perfume and painted on our fingers. Stress from the deferred dreams, the dreams not voiced; stress from the broken promises, the bla-tant lies; stress from always being on the bottom, from never being thought beautiful, from always being taken for granted, taken advantage of; stress from being a black women in white America....

I have quoted this at length because it reveals how a conscious-ness about the social basis of black women's distress is linked to a lay therapeutic—one that stands in opposition to medicalization. Moreover, it stands in sharp contrast to the experiences of FMS sufferers who, in desperation, search for a biomedical answer and a biomedical name for their unexplainable constellations of distress. In other words, part of the cultural disposition of many black women may be a tendency toward the *routinization* and *normalization* of pain (broadly defined). This, too, is cap-tured in *The Black Women's Health Book*, in an essay by Bridgett Davis, who speaks to the pain and grief experienced in black communities:

I believe that on some deeper level, black women are used to tragedy. We expect it. Death is not a stranger to our lives, to our worlds. We've lost our fathers to hypertension and heart attacks, our brothers to frontline battles in American wards, our husbands and lovers to black-on-black crime or police brutality and our sons to drug-laced streets or upstate prisons. All this while grappling with the stress and burden of all that is black life in America: Babies born to babies, dehumanizing ghettos, inferior schools, low wages, on-the-job racism...the slow but steady death of our people. We are just used to pain (B. Davis 1990: 223).

My intent in quoting these black feminist authors is not to reaffirm the cultural myth that black women have unending strength to suffer their oppression gracefully.[4] However poetic the language in which these ideas are expressed, it is essential to avoid such romanticization (Collins 1991; Wallace 1990). Moreover, it is imperative not to lose sight of the bigger picture with respect to black women's health, namely, that the health disparity between black and white women is decidedly in white women's favor. Indeed, some scholars suggest that the myth of the strong black woman may itself contribute to black women's compromised health insofar as they are encouraged to deny their own needs (Harris-Lacewell 2001). Rather, these writings suggest that, among the ironies of persistent suffering are found cultural dispositions built on the *normalization* of suffering, awareness of the social and economic *causes* of suffering, and, consequently, a local cultural world for endowing suffering with *meaning*.

Perhaps black women produce local cultural accounts of their embodied distress, grounded in their identities as black women. It is possible that this cultural disposition toward stress and suffering may partly account for black women's underrepresentation among those with FMS and other functional somatic syndromes, despite the high levels of stress to which they are exposed.

Some empirical evidence supports the essence of this speculative claim. Several studies find that African American women are less favorably inclined toward exclusively medical explanations for, and treatment of, illness. For example, in their study of rural black women with advanced breast cancer, Holly Matthews and her colleagues (1994) found that these women drew on multiple modes of knowledge to give meaning to their illness experience. Among other things, a number of the women in the study refused to acknowledge or accept the biomedical diagnosis of breast cancer. Moreover, the women evoked local accounts of bodily imbalance to account for their illness. In other words, the meaning of breast cancer to these women was not exclusively, and in some cases not even primarily, based on a biomedical account of breast cancer.

Similarly, a community study comparing black and white women's PMS symptoms and complaints found no difference in the reported severity of symptoms, despite the fact that the use of PMS medical services is almost exclusively a white phenomenon (Stout et al. 1986). In contrast to non-Hispanic white women, African American women also routinely incorporate lay health beliefs, practices, and providers into their prenatal care (Morgan 1996). Finally, in a study of 169 individuals diagnosed with severe and persistent mental illness, Sue Estroff and coworkers. (1991) describe the explanations individuals use to account for themselves as ill. The study found that African American women were not as likely to use biomedical accounts of their symptoms as were white women. Indeed, among women, race was a better predictor of whether an individual defined herself as "mentally ill" than was the level of symptom severity.

Studies also find African Americans, regardless of gender, to be more skeptical toward certain types of medical explanations, procedures, and treatments. For example, African American parents are less likely than non-Hispanic white parents to attribute their children's problems to medically informed views of mental health (Yen et al. 2004); and African Americans are less likely than whites to believe in the potential health benefits of predictive genetic screening and are more fearful about the potential for using such information in discriminatory ways (Peters et al. 2004). It is not simply that blacks generally, or black women in particular, are pulled toward lay medical knowledge more than are their white counterparts; blacks are also more put off by biomedicine. African Americans distrust medical research and the U.S. health care system (Boulware et al. 2003; Byrd and Clayton 2000–2002). The historical legacy of the Tuskegee syphilis study and contemporary evidence shows significant racial disparities in the quality of health care received by white and black Americans. The Institute of Medicine's recently published report, *Unequal Treatment* (Smedley et al. 2003), outlines the multiple and complex factors that result in racial and ethnic minorities receiving lower quality health care than whites.

These pieces of evidence, patched together as they are, suggest a greater reticence on the part of African American women toward the medicalization of their experience as well as the availability of non-medical explanations for their physical and mental distress. Although we cannot say for certain why black women are nearly absent among those with FMS, it is plausible that cultural dispositions toward suffering and the institution of medicine play a part. Moreover, the other side of this admittedly speculative interpretation has implications for white women such as Meredith and Betsy.

The stories of FMS sufferers reveal complex worlds of pain—lives infused with ubiquitous and specific physical, material, and emotional hardship and suffering. Yet, sufferers' inability to recognize the complexity of their distress, or to appreciate the regrettable regularity of women's suffering, leads them to narrate their own distress as disease. Their position of social and economic disadvantage (vis-à-vis more affluent women) exposes them to greater hardship and gives them fewer resources with which to alter the situations that infuse their lives with stress and suffering. At the same time, their inclusion within the dominant white culture blunts their awareness of the social forces giving shape to their suffering and leads them to internalize the prevailing cultural assumption regarding the abnormality of pain.

In sum, both social positions and dispositions (Bourdieu and Wacquant 1992) explain the overrepresentation of white, working- and lower middle-class women among those with FMS. Compared with more affluent white women, they share the dominant cultural expectation of a life free from pain, but they often lack the resources with which to realize that norm. Yet, compared with black and other minority women, they also lack a cultural understanding that normalizes the resulting suffering and gives it social meaning. Within their cultural world, suffering is unexpected and unexplainable, and, therefore, in need of, if not a remedy, at least an explanation. FMS, therefore, is associated with genuine suffering that is rooted in the material conditions of women's lives, but it is also dependent on a disposition in which women see themselves as entitled to painlessness and biomedicine as the route to that entitlement.

Conclusion

The Fibromyalgia Syndrome Story

The fibromyalgia syndrome (FMS) story is, at once, both fascinating and unremarkable. It is a fascinating story from a sociological standpoint because of the multiple forces that came together to facilitate the creation of the diagnostic category and the subsequent social phenomena. Pieces of the FMS story range from large-scale cultural and economic trends down to the subjective experience of suffering and efforts to give meaning to that experience. It is impossible to condense the FMS story into a unified decree and various efforts to do so— "psychogenic rheumatism," "neurochemical disorder," "dysregulation spectrum symptom," "iatrogenic illness"—are all limited in their oversimplification. Indeed, a central aim of this book is to remind us just how multifaceted the story of FMS is—far more than most FMS advocates or detractors acknowledge.

On the other hand, the story of FMS is rather unremarkable if one is looking for spectacular and dramatic events or, in the language of our day, "a smoking gun." The creation of FMS was a complicated, but ultimately unsurprising, outcome of predictable behavior on the part of the key social actors. It is also an unremarkable story given how little has been gained or lost through the creation of FMS. There are no unambiguous beneficiaries of the FMS diagnosis nor are there clear victims.

We can and should approach the FMS story with a clear understanding that medically unexplainable somatic complaints are endemic. The specific symptoms identified as the pillars of FMS—musculoskeletal pain and general fatigue—are among the most common physical ailments reported in the general public (Barsky and Borus 1999). At the risk of making an essentialist claim, pain and fatigue should be understood as fundamental to the human experience. Depression, sleep disturbances, and other common FMS symptoms are also widely prevalent. The complex character of much of this malaise remains beyond the reach of biomedicine's ability to identify a specific organic cause or to provide an effective remedy.

Added to this pervasive malaise is women's heightened somatic distress. Compared with men, women report more physical symptoms, are more likely to evaluate their symptoms as serious, and more likely to seek medical assistance in response to their evaluation. This gender difference in somatic complaints is evident in the specific case of pain. Women report greater pain than men in response to the same level of physical stimulation. When women and men report the same subjective levels of pain, women are more likely to seek medical care and report disability (Yunus 2001). The causes for these differences between men and women pose puzzles so complex as to be unsolvable, even with the most sophisticated biomedical research designs and techniques. Thus, although the reasons remain obscure and open to debate, little doubt exists that women exhibit greater somatic distress than men. Or, to reorient the comparison with women at the center, men exhibit less somatic distress than women. Rather than purport to offer the definitive explanation for what has been a focus of speculation for millennia, I shall simply acknowledge this as a central feature of the FMS story. Any serious investigation into FMS, therefore, must begin with the recognition that its core symptoms are regrettably common companions of everyday life, both in the general public and among women in particular.

This is not to say that FMS is much ado about nothing. Whether common or not, the cumulative experience of chronic pain, fatigue, sleep disturbances, depression, and related symptoms can easily become overwhelming. The women whose stories have been presented in the preceding pages make this abundantly clear. The next piece of the FMS story, therefore, calls for an appreciation of the sufferer's need to make sense of, and manage, her somatic distress. Here, we require an awareness of the cultural dominance of biomedicine, both as a set of beliefs and as an institution. In our society, widely shared and taken-for-granted biomedical principles, metaphors, and ideals provide the dominant framework through which embodied reality is experienced and given meaning. So it is we find ourselves simultaneously suffering and seeking to endow our suffering with meaning in terms of commonly understood biomedical standards. When necessary, we turn to the formal institutions of biomedicine to officially interpret and mediate our suffering. In fact, we do so with great regularity because we assume that biomedicine has the capacity to alter the course of nature and that the "normal" state of nature is the absence of suffering. The union of these assumptions accounts for our cultural refusal to accept even inevitable infirmities (Barsky and Borus 1995).

Thus, to comprehend the story of FMS, we must situate the complexity and commonness of women's somatic complaints within the context of biomedical hegemony and resultant dominant cultural sensibilities that understand suffering as abnormal, anomalous, and alterable. This combination of forces brings women, in far greater numbers than men, into the clinic with a wide range of common, but troubling, symptoms. The real and devastating consequences of women's symptoms bring them back, over and over again. Despite the best efforts of medical practitioners, no objective pathology can be found. The voice of the life world and the voice of the biomedicine, therefore, are at odds. This results in self-mortification and the erosion of all that is taken for granted as women's sense of reality is repeatedly invalidated—all taking place against a backdrop of ideological assumptions concerning women's predilections to star in their self-made dramas.

For decades, rheumatology figured centrally in this cycle of failed medical encounters. As the likely referral for patients in pain, rheumatolgists see a great number of patients, a disproportionate number of them women, with widespread, inexplicable pain. Much of the practice of rheumatology involves managing this vast and persistent residual category of patients with pain of unknown origin. During the late 1970s and 1980s, a small cadre of rheumatolgists set out to extricate a subset of patients who had long been consigned to the residual diagnostic category of psychogenic rheumatism. The efforts of these diagnostic entrepreneurs both acknowledged the suffering of patients and promoted their own professional agendas and ambitions as they created a new field of research and practice in which they were experts. The coming together of a large category of women patients (who were similar only insofar as they had a host of unexplainable symptoms) and a small cadre of rheumatolgists interested in transcending the limitations of existing medical nomenclature led to the diagnostic making of FMS.

Fibromyalgia syndrome is an intellectual abstraction whose original premise was built on the notion that what made the category distinct was its *lack* of organic distinction, setting up a logical quandary from the very beginning. Yet, through the practices and principles of diagnostic research, the diagnostic entrepreneurs tautologically validated a set of subjective criteria to define FMS that, unsurprisingly given their patient pool, reflect a highly feminized idiom of distress. In the process, however, the feminization of the disorder was obscured and the resulting body of FMS research cannot address the disorder's feminization. Hence, the peculiarities behind the diagnostic making of FMS, as well as much of the ensuing debate, highlight the mismatch between the complex nature of women's somatic suffering and the orientation and tools of biomedicine.

Nevertheless, as an intellectual abstraction, FMS is both a practical and effective way of giving meaning to a wide array of common distresses that characterize the lives of many women, which, in turn, explains its contemporary prevalence. This is true from the perspective of the doctor and patient alike. Once the diagnosis was created it could be, and continues to be, readily applied, despite widespread medical skepticism. Various commentators have addressed the multiple aspects of the doctor-patient relationship that encourage diagnosing a patient's distressing condition, even when no fully satisfactory diagnosis is available (Barsky and Borus 1995; Barsky and Borus 1999; Freidson 1971; Rosenberg 1997). As a representation of the patient's suffering and the physician's mastery, diagnoses legitimatize both parties and the doctor-patient relationship itself.

Moreover, what we might call the diagnostic imperative is even more pronounced when women patients are involved. For example, in her book *Power Under the Microscope*, Kathy Davis (1988) describes the ways in which medical encounters reclassify women's diffuse physical complaints around menstruation and menopause into biomedical syndromes. On one side are women patients who seek physicians' help with their somatic complaints and, on the other, are physicians who feel an obligation to help their patients. According to Davis, one option would be to use the medical encounter simply to hear women out. Physicians could listen to women and confirm that, although their complaints are indeed unpleasant, they are nevertheless common and not indicative of a discrete medical condition. But physicians are trained to take action and patients want something to be done on their behalf. Consequently, as described by Davis, when women use the clinic to give voice to their physical complaints, physicians respond by framing those complaints as medical syndromes out of a sense of obligation to and concern for their patients.

Davis' account of premenstrual syndrome (PMS) and menopausal deficiency contains many of the same dynamics that result in the routine application of FMS. However, what particularly comes to light in the case of FMS is that, when the clinic is used as a forum simply to hear women out, women sufferers feel discredited and demeaned. In contrast, when they hear a diagnosis, they feel affirmed and validated. Charged by cultural beliefs concerning their irrationality, women's search for illness meaning and the burdens of failed medical encounters seriously erode their sense of self, making the moment of diagnosis a ritualistic passage from being discredited to being authorized. This cathartic and transformative moment suggests that fueling the expansion of the FMS diagnosis are insidious and entrenched gender inequalities and ideologies that dictate how clinical scripts are read and heard by the players in the clinical encounter.

Beyond serving the immediate needs of the clinical encounter, the moment of diagnosis also launches the moral career of the FMS sufferer—that is, it initiates a new self-constructive process, including a new cognitive schema through which the sufferer can give order and coherence to all that she has been experiencing. An especially important step in this career is engagement with the FMS self-help community and its shared narrative. Through the FMS self-help narrative, sufferers develop a cognitive framework for making sense of their particular distress. Because of its permissive boundaries, the FMS narrative logically incorporates more and more of everyday life within its purview. At the same time, it facilitates a sense of affiliation with others—an illness identity—on the basis of shared suffering that ranges from the mundane to the profound. The outcome is the reification of FMS; it is experienced as a real and natural entity rather the product of human activity. Few sufferers fully escape the formation of an FMS illness identity in an era where mass media health resources, products, and technologies are ever-present features of the cultural landscape.

Here, we pick up another important piece in the FMS story, namely the union between suffering and the market economy. Without calling into question the goodwill and compassion of doctors, clinics, authors, publishers, conference and workshop organizers, and webmasters, some have an economic stake in FMS. Recognized authorities in the field of FMS research not only secure and advance their medical careers through this line of research, but also avail themselves of consulting fees, speaking fees, and profitable side ventures (e.g., royalties from the production of self-help books and videos). Although it is easy to accuse those who promote the diagnosis of entrepreneurial behavior, professional ambitions are also realized through criticizing FMS. Advocates accuse critics of making careers out of their published disavowals of the diagnosis and insinuate that they work as henchmen for the insurance industry to deny sufferers medical and disability compensation (White 2004). These various conflicts of interest highlight the impossibility for even the well-intentioned to stand outside of the market economy that informs, shapes, and structures our society at large and into which we have cast our health care system. I would be foolish not to acknowledge that I, too, am enmeshed in this process.

Other economic interests are woven into the FMS story. Advertisements from a glossy magazine exclusively for FMS sufferers, *Fibromyalgia AWARE*, attest to the various market niches sufferers represent. The magazine's pages are filled with advertisements for common FMS prescription and over-the-counter medications, nutritional supplements and vitamins created just for those with FMS, pillows and cushions to improve the sleep and comfort of FMS sufferers, lawyers specializing in post-traumatic fibromyalgia, and an FMS treatment clinic that, as the ad points out, accepts Blue Cross and Blue Shield. In addition to many best-selling books and videos, dozens, if not hundreds, of .com sites for fibromyalgia sufferers provide a world of buying opportunities. Sufferers can buy FMS T-shirts, handbags, coffee mugs, and posters from any number of different support groups and organizations at any number of different online sites. Surrounded by a market economy, sufferers seek to purchase solutions for, as well as representations of, their illness and, in the process, become consumers of FMS goods and services.

Sociologists argue that a defining feature of contemporary capitalist society is the crafting of identities through particular patterns and practices of consumption (Giddens 1991). A thread that runs through the FMS story is the consumerist impulse that assumes we can purchase both product solutions for our troubles and products of selfhood. The construction of an FMS illness identity conflates with a type of consumerism, ranging from shopping for a "fibro-friendly" doctor to the more ambitious and elusive projects of self-understanding and, as such, is exemplary of how the self is constituted via consumption more generally. It also raises questions about the role of the market economy in shaping illness identities by promoting diagnoses and their related industries.

Still other economic forces are at play in the FMS story. It is important, for example, to address how the organizational imperatives and dynamics of managed care contributed to the diagnostic making and expansion of FMS. Patients with unexplainable symptoms are costly and health care organizations necessarily erect barriers to limit their utilization of services. However, Barksy and Borus (1995: 1931) argue that these barriers only lead patients to "express their 'disease' in more urgent and exaggerated terms in order to gain access to the physician." Add to this the fact that patients in prepaid systems have little financial disincentive to seek more and more care and, consequently, many will do so. What is more, sympathetic physicians and other health care providers find that a diagnosis is a helpful "make-do" or "work-around" for getting their patients particular resources within the constraints of managed care. In the case of FMS, organizational efforts to limit patients' access appear to have backfired, introducing new forces that pushed toward greater utilization of health care services, and encouraged the creation and widespread application of a new diagnostic category. It therefore could be argued that the managed care environment inadvertently encouraged the creation and spread of

FMS. Parenthetically, it is likely that these same dynamics also underlie the rise of other contested diagnostic classifications.

We might note, however, that FMS could still turn out to managed care's financial advantage. It has been suggested that diagnosing somatic patients when they first seek medical assistance can reduce costs by reducing the number of expensive (and unnecessary) diagnostic tests, referrals to specialists, and surgeries (Goldenberg 1999). Insofar as the standard treatment protocol for FMS entails prescribing anti-depressants and encouraging cardiovascular exercise and patient education (Goldenberg et al. 2004), it is possible that the costs associated with managing these patients could be dramatically reduced and controlled through early diagnosis. This matter is still under investigation (White et al. 2002). It is, however, not inconceivable that managed care organizations could put the FMS diagnosis (along with other functional somatic diagnoses) to use as part of their cost containing agendas.

Another important factor in the FMS story is the political climate of the 1980s and thereafter. This period is characterized by sharp cutbacks in the welfare state and the effects of these cutbacks have been most pronounced on women with children (Hays 2003; Mink 2002; Seccombe 1999). American exceptionalism—the tendency to let markets rather than the state provide basic services to citizens—has long made the material well-being of less affluent members of society vulnerable to political and economic trends. Harsh cutbacks in recent decades have created a climate in which one of the only ways to make a worthy claim on the ever-less-generous welfare state is to do so on the basis of a medical diagnosis. Demands on the state by citizens, workers, or even mothers are less politically viable, driving more and more individuals to frame their needs and demands as medical.

Other demands have also become simultaneously medicalized and depoliticized. For example, in the early twenty-first century, we find ourselves debating the scientific merits of "repetitive strain injuries," which, although serious, stand in for larger political demands about the rights of workers to exercise control of their work conditions. Consider also Gulf War Syndrome (GWS). GWS is but the latest attempt to have the suffering and sacrifice of combat service recognized medically when it has been denied politically. GWS is of particular interest to us here because it represents the exception to the rule: it is the only contemporary functional somatic syndrome in which men significantly predominate. GWS, therefore, can be read as a male version of the story hitherto told. It too is story in which complex suffering resists orthodox biomedical interpretation and yet demands a diagnostic voice. As with FMS, GWS highlights a resolve on the part of sufferers to have their anguish recognized in a cultural milieu where medicine is perceived either as the best or the only avenue for such recognition. Across a variety of social contexts, diagnoses, thus, have become a key form of political and social capital. In this regard, FMS is but one example of the greater trend in contemporary society in which suffering and disempowerment seek medical diagnoses as possible avenues of recognition and relief.

From what we might call the political economy of the body down to the phenomenology of everyday life, these are some of the many pieces in the complex and overdetermined FMS story. In large measure, therefore, FMS is but a chapter in a larger story about the character, interpretation, and experience of suffering in modern society.

The Social Construction of FMS and Its Future

In this book I have argued that FMS is a socially constructed syndrome that gives meaning to a broad range of distress and suffering that characterizes the lives of many women. But what does it mean to call FMS socially constructed? It means that, as it currently exists, FMS is an intellectual abstraction created through social processes. The diagnostic criteria were tautologically constructed and they remain subjectively determined and inexactly and inconsistently applied. No convincing evidence indicates that the symptoms that are gathered under this diagnostic label have any coherence as a discrete and unitary condition. Instead, considerable evidence shows that FMS is a very large conceptual tent under which many dissimilar types of symptoms can be located and that these symptoms are widespread, in general, and particularly common among women.

Calling FMS a socially constructed syndrome, however, does not necessarily deny the *realness* or physicality of the symptoms that are given this label. After listening to women's FMS stories, it is clear to me that their suffering is *real:* their quality of life is constantly eroded and they would do almost anything to be well. Although I am confident that the diagnostic label of FMS is a social construction, that label might, in fact, represent a number of things that are very real indeed. The socially constructed meanings that mediate our experience of a disorder or condition can be overly simplistic, flawed, or distorted, but that does not mean that the symptoms that comprise the disorder have no physiological basis or that they would cease to exist in the absence of a specific diagnosis. Instead, some things can be *both* socially constructed *and* physiologically real; this may, in fact, prove to be the case for FMS.

Some say that eventually, after we collect enough data, the FMS debate will be resolved. At some point, we will have enough well-designed clinical studies to be able to determine, once and for all, if FMS is a "real" disease and, if so, what causes it and what remedies are effective in its treatment. I do not share this opinion. It seems unlikely that the FMS story will end so simply, given its multifaceted and winding plot thus far.

Partly because of the complexity of the FMS story, I have made every effort to listen to, and honor, women's subjective accounts of their illness. Nevertheless, their subjective reports of sickness are not, in and of themselves, evidence of a discrete and bounded objective disease. One must not blur this distinction. We live in an era when scientific reason, in principle, is culturally authoritative, but as Wendy Kaminer (1999) persuasively argues, we also live in a time wherein subjectivity has become sacrosanct and personal testimony stands in for evidence of objective realities. In other words, a type of subjectivist evangelicalism permeates our culture. There are evangelical FMS sufferers and they will read this book as invalidating. Even though individuals diagnosed with FMS are truly suffering and it is imperative that we acknowledge and respond to their distress, no compelling evidence indicates that they share an "it" (i.e., a discrete and unified medical condition). Their subjective experience of distress no more confirms such a biophysical entity than the absence of biophysical evidence disconfirms their suffering or proves that it is psychosomatic.

Then again, it seems highly implausible that the majority of individuals whose condition is diagnosed as FMS cause their own symptoms (either consciously or unconsciously). Ample clinical research finds a normal psychological profile in many FMS sufferers, and, although they do have high rates of depression and anxiety, many functioning citizens walk our streets similarly distressed. In short, there is no persuasive evidence that individuals with FMS, as a group, are suffering under the weight of major emotional and mental instability. The crucial point to keep in mind is that the tremendous heterogeneity in types of distress captured under the label of FMS also guarantees that sufferers will represent a very heterogeneous population in terms of emotional and mental health.

By extension, a solution to FMS is not likely to result from an increased recourse to mental health referrals, although such consultation may help FMS sufferers in the same way that it can help anyone dealing with the devastating loss that chronic illness brings. Nor, however, is it likely that FMS sufferers will suddenly improve once the illness behavior-inspiring diagnosis is dismantled, as many of the most vocal opponents propose. Sufferers act in response to their distress, not to the label for their distress, although I have demonstrated how the diagnostic label aids in a particular organization of that distress and bestows on it particular meaning. It is also improbable that biomedicine will discover the "magic bullet" that remedies the suffering of women diagnosed with FMS. Judging from the available research evidence, it seems overwhelmingly likely that FMS sufferers share a multiplicity of diffuse and troubling symptoms that are sufficiently different in their nature and etiology that no single therapy is likely to be effective in their overall treatment.

Despite this fact, the tendency for FMS sufferers to promote an exclusively biomedical account of their distress makes all the sense in the world. A biomedical diagnosis and organic account of one's suffering offers both cultural legitimacy and hope of remedy. But efforts to medicalize a broad range of women's distresses under FMS puts all the eggs, so to speak, in the biomedical basket. Even if the improbable transpires and some neurochemical abnormality should come to be associated unequivocally with FMS, what would this tell us about the complexity of suffering that FMS represents? Would such a neurochemical abnormality be the cause or the effect of women's somatic distress? Despite concerted efforts to demonstrate the contrary, the broad range and complex character of women's suffering currently housed under the FMS diagnosis resists being meaningfully captured within the biomedical model.

At this juncture, one might be expected to present the standard social science and feminist critique of biomedicine and demand that it be more attentive to the social forces that shape women's health. Certainly, I have pointed out these limitations throughout this book. But this is not my charge. The problem is not just the need for biomedicine to become more sociological, multidimensional, and intellectually creative. In fact, there is something unsettling about biomedicine's intellectual and jurisdictional expansion into worlds outside its purview. "Biopsychosocial" accounts are now the rage and there is finally hope that the narrow biological focus of biomedicine is adapting to the complex character of women's health. One can point to a small handful of biopsychosocial studies (e.g., Barsky and Borus 1999) that incorporate social and psychological factors in a sophisticated and insightful way. In the main, however, biological facts remain the principal currency in the institution of biomedicine, and most attempts to stir in "psychosocial" variables are poorly done, undervalued, and may, in fact, represent new forms of medical imperialism, surveillance, and control.

It is not simply the assumptions of biomedicine that need altering. We must become less dependent on biomedicine for making sense of our lives and our suffering. We need to be more sociological, multidimensional, and intellectually creative ourselves. We need to politicize the ways that social and economic forces impact the well-being of those who are relatively disempowered, knowing full well that those forces and their effects cannot be captured biomedically. We need to produce a public narrative that makes sense of pain and distress as grounded in the everyday fabric of women's (and men's) lives and that directs our energies toward the search for solutions beyond the realm of biomedicine. If the extensive publicity and debate surrounding FMS can help move us closer to these goals, then perhaps the story of FMS will prove to be a pivotal episode in the greater quest to make sense of human suffering and to find more effective solutions to that portion of human anguish that is caused or amplified by the social conditions in which we live.

Appendix A. The Fibromyalgia Syndrome Biomedical Literature

There were 1,120 English language fibromyalgia publications between 1975 and the end of 2000. This figure is based on a *MEDLINE* search conducted February 7, 2001. It is possible that a small number of publications for 2000 were omitted from my analysis, given that *MEDLINE* indexing is not an instantaneous process for all journals. This is especially true for international journals.

A title, rather than keyword search, was conducted on both fibrositis and fibromyalgia. Based on two pilot samples of fifty abstracts each (one generated using a title search and one using a keyword search), the title search did not include any abstracts or articles whose substantive focus was not fibromyalgia, whereas the keyword search included four such articles. Consequently, using a title search made the laborious task of coding publication abstracts more manageable by eliminating a large number of abstracts summarizing articles not primarily focused on fibrositis or fibromyalgia. I recognize that this strategy excluded publications without fibrositis or fibromyalgia in the title, although the substantive focus was indeed fibrositis or fibromyalgia. This strategy likely excluded only a small number of relevant articles, and, more importantly, not in a manner that would systematically bias the data's representativeness.

The main logic for using a title rather than keyword search was to avoid the problems of retrospective reclassification done through *MEDLINE* indexing. I was interested in research that was self-consciously about fibrositis or fibromyalgia at the time it was conducted, not research that was retrospectively labeled by *MEDLINE* as related to fibromyalgia or fibrositis. If authors titled their publication using the term fibrositis or fibromyalgia, then I knew they were consciously identifying themselves with this area of biomedical research. No other search feature in *MEDLINE* (e.g., mesh or keyword search) offered this assurance. I first became aware of this problem when I tried to find the first publication using the term "fibromyalgia." I discovered that articles published several decades before the term fibromyalgia was ever used had been retrospectively keyword-indexed as fibromyalgia articles.

The first stage of analysis included coding all 1,120 publication abstracts. Articles were coded as research articles, review articles, or editorials. Additionally, articles were coded in terms of primary focus. For example, articles were identified as association or causation articles, diagnostic articles, treatment articles, epidemiological articles, or articles involving disability or quality of life issues. Finally, the substantive focus was further coded (e.g., type of treatment being studied; the causal model being studied) as well as the basic research findings (e.g., a positive or negative treatment outcome; evidence supporting or failing to support the causal model.)

Table A.1 summarizes the focus of research articles. Of the 627 research articles, nearly half explore factors associated with FMS, possibly causally, whereas more than 15 percent evaluated treatment protocols for FMS.

Table A.1. Research Article Focus, 1975–2000

Focus	Number of articles	Percent of articles
Causality/Association	292	44.6
Treatment/Evaluation	97	15.5
Co-morbidity	59	9.4
Measuring disability in FMS	47	7.5
Measuring pain in FMS	35	5.6
Diagnostic evaluation	22	3.5
Children and FMS	17	2.7
Epidemiology	11	1.8
Clinical overview	5	.8
Other	42	6.7
TOTAL	627	100.0

Table A.2.   Association or Causation Research Articles, 1975–2000

Substantive focus	Number of articles	Percent of articles
Neurobiological	100	34.2
Muscle pathology	40	13.7
Psycho-behavioral	39	13.4
Sleep abnormality	27	9.2
Postviral/immune	22	7.5
Cardiovascular/fitness	16	5.5
Breast implants/female reproductive body	7	2.4
Other	41	14.0
TOTAL	292	100.0

Table A.2 illustrates the substantive focus of research articles exploring factors associated with FMS, including possible casual factors.

Given the scattered focus of research publications, forty-one of the association or causation research articles could not be coded into a category constituting more than 1 or 2 percent of the total association or causation research articles. For this reason, nearly twenty categories, each with only a few articles, were collapsed into the category "other" in Table A.2.

Appendix B. The Interviews

The Sample

Thirty women and four men diagnosed with fibromyalgia syndrome (FMS) were interviewed for this study. Twenty-six women and all the men were asked to reflect on their FMS experience using questions designed to encourage narration. Six women participated in a focus group interview concerning the role of self-help books in their FMS experience. Of these six women, two were among the twenty-six women interviewed more broadly.

Fifteen women were interviewed after they responded to a flyer distributed at a FMS conference co-sponsored by the Arthritis Foundation and a university-based fibromyalgia research organization. The flyer requested research participants for a study into the social and cultural aspects of FMS. The conference, held in a metropolitan area, was attended by more than 300 individuals, including many who had traveled a considerable distance. The remaining women were contacted through local FMS support groups located in diverse communities. Three of the men signed up to participate in the study through local support groups; one did so through the aforementioned conference.

The primary strengths of this sample are its nonclinical base, its geographical representation, and its inclusion of members as well as nonmembers of FMS support groups. The limitations of clinic- or patient-based research have been well articulated: Usually, patient populations are more severely ill than community populations and they often differ significantly in terms of key social variables, including class, level of education, and race or ethnic background. The sample in this study includes women from nine different cities of varying sizes, including a large metropolitan area, a mid-sized university town, and several small semirural communities. These cities are in two adjoining states. Six different support groups were used as sites for participant recruitment. Many of those contacted via support groups, however, attended only one or two meetings or were only marginally involved in the support group's activities. Moreover, of those individuals contacted via the aforementioned conference, many were not active in a FMS support group. The women were split equally between regular support group attendees and those who had never or rarely attended a support group. The men were contacted through three different support groups in two different cities, but none of them identified themselves as active support-group attendees. Three men reported having attended support group meetings only one or two times, whereas one reported slightly more involvement.

Most research suggests that men make up less than 10 percent of those with FMS. The explicit focus of this project is women with FMS. Nevertheless, it seemed advisable to interview a few men, although such a small number of interviews clearly cannot yield generalizable findings nor is it sufficient to test for intersex variation. Because men are on the margins of (although not absent from) the population of those who suffer from FMS, information gathered through interviews with them is presented mainly as endnotes. This seemed the best way to capture their marginal location within the phenomenon of FMS without ignoring their presence altogether.

Social Characteristics of Participants

This section presents summary characteristics of the twenty-six women who participated in the in-depth semistructured interviews. All twenty-six women were white. They ranged in age from twenty-eight to sixty-five years, with a mean age of forty-eight. The mean educational level for the women in this sample was less than thirteen years. Three women did not graduate from high school, eleven had a high school diploma only, eight had some trade or college courses without a degree, and four women had a bachelor's degree. Demographically, this sample compares closely in terms of race or ethnicity, age, and education to the distributions reported in previous community prevalence studies, suggesting that it is not unrepresentative of the distribution of FMS in the population at large (White et al. 1999; Wolfe et al. 1995).

Comparable information for the men can be summarized briefly. All were white and ranged in age from thirty-three to forty-six years, with a mean age of forty. Two of the men had high school diplomas, one attended two years of college, and one had a masters degree; men had an average of fourteen years of schooling.

Semistructured Interviews

Interviews, which were semistructured, lasted between one and three hours, with the average interview length of one hour and thirty minutes. Twenty-four of the interviews with women were conducted face-to-face; two were conducted over the telephone; all but two interviews took place at the interviewee's home (or mother's home in the case of the two mother-daughter interviews). All interviews were conducted by either the author or research assistant, Natalie Boero. Ms. Boero conducted nine interviews, although the author also spoke with each of these nine women either by telephone or face to face.

Interviews were tape-recorded and transcribed verbatim, excluding repetitious or unnecessary phrases (e.g., "you know," "like"). Three participants did not consent to being taped, and their interviews were transcribed from extensive interviewer notes. Biographical details were altered slightly to ensure confidentiality. No changes were made that significantly altered the essence of the interview. Several women requested a copy of their interview transcriptions and those requests were honored. Interviews were analyzed using qualitative text analysis software.

All four men were interviewed face to face, but one did not consent to being tape-recorded. The average interview for men was nearly an hour and fifty minutes, although the range was dramatic: one interview lasted three hours, whereas another was completed in forty-five minutes.

The first question asked in the interview was, "Can you tell me about when you first started experiencing symptoms you now understand as being related to your fibromyalgia?" This question was designed to encourage interviewees to narrate their FMS story from its beginning to the present. Many interviews did proceed along these lines and, after an hour or so of narration, the interviewee had managed to address all the questions on the interview schedule. When specific information was not provided in this free-flowing narrative form, the interviewee was asked questions directly from the interview schedule (see below).

In addition to describing when they first started experiencing FMS symptoms, interviewees were also asked how their symptoms impacted their everyday lives and how they changed over time, as well as what type of medical care they sought and received. Specific questions were asked about when and how their condition was diagnosed as FMS, including who had diagnosed the condition, how it was diagnosed, and how the diagnosis affected their illness experience. Interviewees were also asked questions about their involvement in the FMS self-help or mutual support communities, and about disability and disability compensation. Basic demographic information on age, race or ethnicity, occupation, education, and family status was also collected

Although questions were designed to encourage narrative responses, a semistructured format was used to balance the principles of reliability and validity. This ensured that responses could be compared across interviews, but also allowed individuals to identify the sequence of salient events in their own FMS experience. The semistructured format also ensured that questions of substantive and theoretical interest would be addressed.

Focus Group Interview

The focus group interview took place at the support group leader's home during a regular meeting. As with many FMS support groups, this particular group recommends that its members read *Fibromyalgia and Chronic Myofascial Pain Syndrome: A Survival Manual,* by far the most widely read FMS self-help book on the market. Six women participated in this interview; the organizing questions were as follows:

1.   What did you think the first time you read *A Survival Manual*?
2.   In what ways, if any, did the book help you make sense of or help you deal with your fibromyalgia?
3.   How well does the book describe your own experience with FMS?
4.   What other FMS self-help books have you read? How have they helped you make sense of your FMS?

Although the focus group questions were specifically about self-help literature, participants also provided details about their general FMS experience. As noted, two women who participated in the focus group were included in the larger sample, but the remaining four are excluded from the sample parameters.

Semistructured Interview Schedule

The specific questions listed as bullets were used as probes if the interviewee did not volunteer this information in her or his narrative answers.

1. Can you tell me about when you first started experiencing symptoms you now understand as being related to your fibromyalgia?
    • What were your symptoms like when they first began?

- Is there anything you can identify as triggering these symptoms?
- Generally, how would you describe your health history before your FMS?
- How did your symptoms impact your daily life?
2. Can you tell me how your FMS symptoms have changed over time?
3. When did you first seek medical attention for your symptoms?
   - What type of medical insurance did you have?
   - How did various health care practitioners respond to your symptoms?
   - How effective was the health care you received?
   - How frequently did you seek health care?
   - What types of medical tests were done?
4. Can you provide a general timeline of health care professionals you have seen in relation to your fibromyalgia symptoms?
   - What type of medical insurance did you have?
   - How did various health care practitioners respond to your symptoms?
   - How effective was the health care you received?
   - How frequently did you seek health care?
   - What types of medical tests were done?
5. Can you tell me about when you were first diagnosed with fibromyalgia? (If the answer to question 4 already addressed this point, ask: Can you give me any more details about when you were first diagnosed with fibromyalgia that you have not already provided?)
   - What tests were done (American College of Rheumatology [ACR] tender point examination)?
   - Who was your doctor or health care practitioner (specialty)?
   - Had you ever heard of FMS when you were diagnosed?
   - How did being diagnosed make you feel?
6. How did being diagnosed impact your experiences with fibromyalgia, or what was the overall impact of your diagnosis on your experience with FMS?
   - Did it shape how you felt about your symptoms?
   - How did your family respond to your diagnosis?
   - How did it shape the types of medical care you received?
   - Did your diagnosis prompt you to find out (more) about FMS?
   - Did your diagnosis prompt you to become involved in a support group?
7. This next question follows from what you have already told me, but I have not asked it directly. Thinking about your daily experiences before and after your diagnosis, what are the main or central differences?

8. Can you tell me about your experiences with fibromyalgia support resources, for example, self-help books, support groups, other fibromyalgia organizations, and Internet sites?

Books

- Have you read any, and what have you learned from them?
- Which books have you liked most and why? (SHOW LIST)

Support Groups

- Have you attended support group meetings? How long have you participated and what has been the nature of your participation?
- How important has the participation been to you in terms of shaping your experiences with fibromyalgia?

Internet

- Do you use Internet resources? What kind of information have you received and how helpful would you say the sites have been?

9. Do you consider fibromyalgia a disability? Have you applied for or do you receive any disability compensation related to your FMS? Can you explain that process?
10. I want to end with a few questions concerning basic demographic information.
    - What is your age?
    - What is your highest level of education?
    - What is your (was your) occupation?
    - What is your current marital status?
    - Do you have children? How many?
11. In closing, is there anything else that you can think of that we have not yet addressed that is important in terms of understanding your experience with FMS?
12. Do you have any questions for me?

Notes

Introduction

1. Starlanyl and Copeland (1996) popularized the phrase "Irritable Every-thing Syndrome" in their best-selling self-help book, but this phrase was used earlier used by Smythe (1985) in a chapter in the *Textbook of Rheumatology*.

2. Some medical sociologists make hard-core social constructionists claims (e.g., that *nothing* exists outside of our socially and historically bound mental constructions). This is not the perspective used here. Instead, I have drawn on several clear-headed accounts of social constructionism, including Phil Brown (1995) and Eliot Freidson (1971). For example, Phil Brown (1995: 37) offers the following helpful claim: "I cannot see that an appreciation of actual condi-tions must automatically prevent us from grasping the social construction of the definition and treatment."

3. Even if "human thought arises, and operates ... in a definite social milieu," explains Mannheim (1936: 80), "[w]e need not regard it as a source of error that all thought is so rooted."

4. I have cited Hacking here even though he is highly critical of social construc-tionism as an explanatory framework. I have done so because I have benefited from his clear reasoning on this point—that something can be both real *and* socially constructed. I disagree with Hacking that social constructionist perspec-tives *necessarily* reproduce a false binary: an entity is either real (and therefore has an entirely biophysical basis) or socially constructed (and therefore has no biophysical basis whatsoever).

5. The definition/timeline of biomedicine used in this book differs from that presented in Clarke et al. (2003). Strictly speaking, biomedicine emerged with the union of medical practice and the lab-based life sciences in the decades brack-eting the turn of the twentieth century. Clarke et al. restrict the use of the term "biomedicine" to apply to more recent historical developments. As they detail masterfully, processes of biomedicalization are now so extensive as to represent historically important social and cultural changes as compared with the earlier era. However, these changes do not represent a fundamental historical break

211

with, but rather the acceleration of, trends that have their roots in the institutionalization of biomedicine circa 1880–1920.

6. In a recent book, Sally Satel (2000) argues that feminists complaints about women being "the second class medical citizen" are unfounded. Satel marshals considerable evidence showing that women have not been systematically excluded from medical research nor have women's health issues taken a back seat in terms of federal funding and medical research attention. I trust that her facts on these points are roughly accurate; however, this is not the same concern advanced here with respect to woman as "biomedical other." Rather the point here is that, at the conceptual level, medicine has historically conflated universality and masculinity. It is this medical assumption that facilitates the medicalization of women's normal physicality and which has historically framed women's illnesses principally in terms of their reproductive bodies. These assumptions can misdirect medical research by focusing excessive attention on women's reproductive physiology in clinical research when women's reproductive physiology is not at play.

Chapter 1

1. The ARA became the ACR in 1988 after severing its association with the Arthritis Foundation (an alliance forged in 1965). The ACR represents rheumatolgists as well as associated health professionals who treat rheumatic patients (i.e., it is not limited to physicians).

2. Hip and joint replacements, one of the most dramatic recent improvements in the treatment of rheumatic disease, fall within the jurisdiction of orthopedic surgeons.

3. One can think of the following crude taxonomy of medical specialization (along with a few examples): population-based (geriatrics and pediatrics); technology-based (radiology, surgery, and anesthesiology); organ- or system-based (dermatology, gastroenterology, and hematology); and disease-based (oncology and infectious disease). This is not a sophisticated taxonomy nor a complete listing of fields (and subfields) of specialization, but it does clarify the point being made here. Even as geriatric physicians encounter a wide range of illnesses and diseases, their patient population (the elderly) functions as the field's organizing rationale. Although radiologists see patients with a wide range of disorders, they encounter all of their patients through radiographic technologies. A specialty needs only one conceptual rationale. Rheumatology was established to treat disorders of the musculoskeletal system, but what brings most patients to rheumatologists is pain, regardless of its nature, and so what could have served as the principal conceptual justification for the field is not well observed. Perhaps other specialties (and subspecialties) are also only loosely conceptually coherent or integrated, but at least they have less-permeable bases for defining their terrain than does rheumatology.

In practice, pain has become the conceptual justification for rheumatology. The only other field of medical specialization justified on the basis of symptomatic expression is psychiatry—a field whose low status relative to other specialties is well recognized. This makes sense given that symptoms are not the "stuff" of biomedical science. It also explains why both psychiatry and rheumatology (in the case of FMS) look to neurology for their scientific legitimacy.

4. The first classificatory nomenclature for rheumatic disease was established in 1941. It was formally revised in 1963 and over the years new diseases were added to bring the classification up to date. In 1941 the ARA adopted nomenclature with nine rheumatic disease classifications and no subclassifications (Smyth et al. 1985: 74). By 1963, there were nearly a hundred diagnoses or conditions organized into thirteen rheumatic disease classification categories (Blumberg et al. 1964).

5. Charles Rosenberg's phrase, "framing disease," is used at various places in this book in recognition of the general claim that disease comes to be known and understood through historically and culturally specific classificatory and explanatory schemes.

6. Brown identifies four different types of conditions and their corresponding definitions. There are medically accepted conditions with biomedical definitions (routinely defined conditions); medically accepted conditions that lack biomedical definitions (contested definitions); conditions that are not medically accepted but which have a biomedical definition (medicalized definitions); and conditions that are not medically accepted and also lack a biomedical definition (potentially medicalized definitions). Brown identifies chronic fatigue syndrome as a medicalized definition. Whereas most physicians question the legitimacy of the condition (i.e., they question its organic basis), a medical definition is routinely applied. By extension, using Brown's terminology, FMS is also a medicalized definition.

7. Fibromyalgia syndrome was initially called "fibrositis syndrome" by clinician researchers and, for a time, both terms were widely used. The generally accepted term for the disorder is now fibromyalgia syndrome. To avoid confusion and wordiness, the acronym FMS is used to denote both fibrositis syndrome and fibromyalgia syndrome.

8. An earlier version of this chapter in *Arthritis and Allied Conditions* was written by rheumatologist Wallace Graham. Smythe took a sharply different position from Graham, however, by arguing that there was a clear boundary between fibrositis and psychogenic rheumatism. Graham offered a more nuanced account of the disorder, suggesting that it was a complex syndrome, with both organic and psychological origins.

9. Multiple tender points were only one aspect of the fibrositis criteria proposed in Smythe's 1972 chapter in *Arthritis and Allied Conditions*. He listed obligatory criteria including a minimum of three months of subjective aching and stiffness, local tender points in multiple areas, and normal laboratory and radiographic tests. He also listed minor symptoms that were not necessarily present in all patients, including chronic fatigue, emotional distress, poor sleep, and morning stiffness. He modified these criteria for a revised version of this chapter in 1979, at which time he specified the number of tender points (twelve of fourteen tender points) and removed emotional distress from the list of possible minor symptoms.

10. This statement is an oversimplification, but not inaccurate. From the first clinical testing of FMS diagnostic criteria up through the ACR study, researchers compared patients with fibromyalgia and controls using different criteria for fibromyalgia. Some researchers required their patients with fibromyalgia to have several associated symptoms, such as fatigue and morning stiffness, whereas others did not. The only shared criterial feature in *all* definitions of fibromyalgia during the 1980s and in the ACR study, however, was multiple tender points. For example, the sixteen participating research centers contributing patients to the ACR study used different FMS criteria. Each center was asked to use its "usual method of diagnosis." The one, shared criterial feature across all centers was the presence of multiple tender points. It is hardly surprising, therefore, that multiple tender points proved to be so effective at discriminating between patients and controls, because it was the only diagnostic criterion shared by all the sixteen centers that contributed subjects to the study's patient pool.

11. The numbers and figures used in this section are based on publications through 2000. I have, however, added citations to more recent published research, editorials, and letters in my descriptions of the current state of knowledge about FMS.

12. See Appendix A for details concerning the *MEDLINE* search used for this study. Excluded from Figure 1.1 are articles that did not have a published abstract ($n = 94$).

13. Although it is widely accepted that FMS does not have an immune component, the debate concerning the related disorder of chronic fatigue syndrome remains somewhat more contentious.

14. Some in the organic camp have appropriated the term "biopsychosocial," but they have done so in ways that distort the original intent proposed by Masi (1998) and others. For example, all that Henirksson (2002: 45) means by the term "biopsychosocial" is that psychological, personality, and social factors "play a role for the total clinical picture." This, of course, is a true statement for any illness whatsoever and, therefore, conceptually vacuous. Henriksson's organic orientation is made fully clear in the following remarks: "There is strong support for the notion that pain and allodynia/hyperalgesia in FMS have an organic cause. ... The permanent changes constitute a disease. There are methods for objectively diagnosing this disease" (Henriksson 2002: 55).

Chapter 2

1. There is also a series of letters addressing the relationship between FMS and silicone breast implants published in *Lancet*, April 19, 1997. Given that my analysis is restricted to research articles, these letters are not counted here. However, the tenor of these letters, in line with the findings from the few published research articles addressing this matter, is a rejection of the relationship between FMS and breast implants.

2. A review article did eventually come out in 2001, written by Muhammad Yunus and published in *Current Rheumatology Reports*, a year after the period encompassed in this study.

3. See Table A.2 in Appendix A for details on the substantive focus in FMS research articles that test various association and causation hypotheses.

4. Women's rates of depression and anxiety disorders are 50 to 100 times greater than men's (Rieker and Bird 2000: 100).

5. It is interesting to note that the sex gap in mortality in the United States appears to be closing. It has fallen slightly since 1970 when it was at a high of 7.7. This is likely the result of a decline in male mortality, not a rise in women's (Kalben 2003).

6. Recent community mental health surveys find gender parity in rates of psychological disorders overall (Rieker and Bird 2000: 100), but women consistently report more emotional and psychological problems than men.

7. Micale (1995) provides a fine and condensed history of the shifts in medical ideas surrounding hysteria. In brief, he suggests that ancient Egyptians, Greeks, and Romans had naturalized conceptions of hysteria that linked women's reproductive physiology to a host of peculiar physical and behavioral symptoms. Thus, despite variations in the theories of hysteria during these three historical periods, all held what Micale calls a "gynecological" conception of the disorder. The next phase in the history of hysteria is marked by the rise of Western Christian civilizations. Between the 5th and 13th centuries, the earlier naturalistic accounts of hysteria were replaced by supernatural accounts (Micale 1995: 20). In short, the hysteric was demonic. The next period in the history of hysteria begins in the 17th century with the rise of neurological theories of disease in general, and of hysteria in particular. This marked a return to a naturalistic account of the condition. The naturalistic or neurological account of hysteria was promoted by Charcot but his views were not widely adopted and by the turn of the 20th century, the next period in the history of hysteria was underway. This period was characterized by the psychologization of hysteria and Sigmund Freud (1856–1939) is the individual most associated with this psychogenic turn.

8. It is a very tricky matter to address the social epidemiology of 19th century disorders (e.g., hysteria and neurasthenia) and even trickier yet to then compare and contrast the social epidemiology of these disorders with the social epidemiology of contemporary patients with CFS or FMS. Nevertheless, exploring the ways the typical hysteric or neurasthenic was like or unlike the average patient with CFS or FMS can be instructive.

Jean-Martin Charcot practiced in an antiquated public hospital for women located in a working-class section of Paris. The hospital, Salpêtrière, was more of a "poorhouse" than a modern clinic. Hundreds of poor, depraved, and demented women were detained rather than treated within the walls of Salpêtrière (Didi-Huberman 2003). Charcot's hysteric patients (ten times more women than men), were women from very modest backgrounds; two thirds were from the working class (Showalter 1997). Although the image of the hysteric that emerged from Charcot's clinic became a part of popular culture, the evidence suggests that, as hysteria spread across Europe and the United States, most of its sufferers were not from comparably modest socioeconomic backgrounds. The large percentage of working-class women hysterics whose condition Charcot diagnosed was likely an artifact of the location and public character of Charcot's clinic. In dramatic contrast, Freud's patients were generally from well-to-do families. Dora, the name Freud gave to his most famous hysteric, was the daughter of a successful textile manufacturer, although it should be noted that Dora, like most of Freud's hysterics, also differed from Charcot's in presenting mundane rather than dramatic symptomology. Dora suffered from a chronic cough, persistent headaches, and depression. It is difficult to say how closely (if at all) the socioeconomic backgrounds of patients seen by these famous physicians mirrored those seen by rank and file practitioners of their times; in general, however, the evidence points to a positive association between middle or upper class status and hysteria (Shorter 1992; Showalter 1997).

Because the nervous exhaustion that characterized neurasthenia was thought triggered principally by mental strain, the relationship between socioeconomic privilege and neurasthenia is more clear-cut. It has been suggested that neurasthenia was often the hysteric diagnosis used by physicians when treating elite women, especially women intellectuals and artists (Showalter 1997). Medical thinking of the time construed mental strain as more deleterious for women than for men because it was more at odds with their nature and the particular demands of the female reproductive body (Newman 1985).

In sum, most of those whose condition was diagnosed as hysteria and neurasthenia in the late 19th and early 20th centuries were white women, primarily from the privileged classes. This was certainly the case in the United States. By comparison, in the United States today, most of those diagnosed with FMS are also white women, but there is a strong *inverse* relationship between FMS and socioeconomic status. It, thus, appears that the class background of those with FMS differs from that of these earlier disorders. This comparison, however, is an uncertain one. In the late 19th and early 20th century in the United States, privileged women would have had greater access to medical care and, therefore, greater access to these diagnoses. In contrast, throughout most of the 20th century access to health care has dramatically expanded. Moreover, today we use fairly sophisticated community studies to determine the prevalence of a condition in the population at large. Because epidemiological studies were rudimentary and rare a century ago, our knowledge of hysteria and neurasthenia is based on the clinical face of these disorders at a time when only a small segment of the population had access to the clinic (again with notable exception of Charcot's hysterics). Thus, the race and class composition of hysteria and neurasthenia sufferers can hardly surprise us.

Despite the problems with these historical comparisons, the gender and racial composition of FMS at the turn of the 21st century (based on both clinical and community studies) does not appear markedly dissimilar from the gender and racial composition of hysteria and neurasthenia at the turn of the 20th century (based primarily on clinical studies). This historical consistency, however, cannot be said for the class of sufferers. At both the community and clinical level, FMS is inversely related to class privilege. Consequently, if we focus on the changing clinical face of these disorders with respect to social class, we can speak to changes across time in who has access to (and the greatest need for) framing their complaints in medical terms. These themes are addressed in greater detail in Chapter 8.

9. In 1979, Smythe noted that tender points, the defining characteristic of fibrositis, were "remarkably constant in location, in patients of varying age, sex, and race" (Smythe 1979: 882).

10. From Betty Friedan's (1963: 20) *The Feminine Mystique*: "Sometimes, she went to the doctor with symptoms she could hardly describe.... A Cleveland doctor called it 'the housewife's syndrome.' "

11. The definition of political correctness (PC) from Princeton University's Wordnet (http://wordnet.princeton.edu/) is the "avoidance of expressions or actions that can be perceived to exclude or marginalize or insult people who are socially disadvantaged or discriminated against" (Cognitive Science Laboratory 2005).

Chapter 3

1. See Appendix B for details about interview questions and sample. The mean age and educational level given are based on twenty-six women who received in-depth interviews and does not incorporate demographic information from four women who participated only in a focus group interview where this information was not collected.

As noted in Appendix B, four men were also interviewed as part of this study. In Chapter 6, I discuss briefly (and with appropriate caveats regarding the small number of cases) certain themes from these interviews and what they suggest about possible gender differences in the experience of FMS. Lest there be any misunderstanding, however, I make no pretence in this study of explicating the FMS experience of the tiny fraction of men who suffer from FMS, nor do I pretend to offer systematic evidence on the similarities and differences in the FMS experiences of men and women. This project focuses on the subjective experiences of *women* whose condition is diagnosed as FMS. Claims regarding the gendered nature of women's FMS experience are based not on statistical comparisons between men and women, but on an interpretative analysis of women's narrative accounts as informed by an extensive body of existing research on gender, gender differences, and the complex link between women's lives and women's health.

2. This is, indeed, a small sample and I have made no effort to make it a scientifically representative or random sample. I do, however, address some of the strengths of this sample, despite its small size, in Appendix B. I primarily recruited subjects from one statewide FMS educational event with an eye to selecting women from different towns of different sizes, as well as women who were both active and not active in self-help groups. These seemed like important variables to take into consideration from a *sociological* perspective. This approach is called "purposive sampling," a technique widely used in the field of sociology.

Any number of possible biases are found in this type of sample. It is possible that the women I interviewed have higher or lower blood pressure, more or less disease severity, and more or less mental health symptoms, to name but a few possibilities, than do women with FMS in general. The same, however, can be said of virtually *every* published clinical study on FMS. Clinical research rarely, if ever, employs true random sampling or addresses the representativeness of its samples. Selection bias occurs in who comes into the clinic and who consents to participate in the studies. Moreover, the number of research subjects in these clinical studies is often as small or smaller than the number of subjects in this study.

For practical reasons, clinical research can rarely aspire to the ideal of representativeness based on random selection, but there are practical methods to minimize the potential bias associated with nonrandom sampling. The same is true in sociology. For the purposes of this study, what matters is that this small sample of women looks demographically like accounts of others suffering from FMS in published population and clinical studies: They are mainly white, middle-aged, and have low levels of education. They may or may not be representative of others who suffer from FMS on any number of other factors, but they are not unrepresentative of those who suffer from FMS in terms of several key variables of interest to sociologists.

3. Themes raised in the formal interviews were also regular themes at support group meetings. I heard similar comments from many different support group participants at several different groups that I attended over a two-year period. Likewise, the narrative similarities were confirmed through countless informal conversations I have had with FMS sufferers over the years. None of the material gathered from these sources is presented here. Nevertheless, these group and informal conversations have contributed to my thinking about FMS and I am grateful to those who shared their FMS experiences with me in these venues.

4. *National Vital Statistics Reports*, Vol. 49, No.12. http://www.cdc.gov/nchs/data/nvsr/nvsr49/nvsr49_12.pdf. January 25, 2005.

5. "Phenomenological philosophy claims to be a philosophy of man in his life-world and to be able to explain the meaning of this life-world in a rigorously scientific manner" (Schutz 1967: 120).

6. Good empirical examples include Bury (1982), Frank (1991; 1995), Good (1994), Kleinman (1988; 1986), and Williams (1984). For a helpful discussion on the theoretical applications of phenomenology to medical sociology, see Turner (1992).

7. In a feminist commentary on Schutz, Dorothy Smith (1987) reminds us of the potentially gendered nature of the everyday life world, arguing that the taken-for-grantedness of many activities, indeed, can be taken for granted by some (mainly men) because the often unseen labor of others (mainly women) makes such taken-for-grantedness possible. Lengermann and Niebrugge (1995) offer another feminist perspective on Schutz.

8. The notion of civil death suggested here parallels that described by Erving Goffman in his account of asylum inmates. The civil death described by those who suffer from FMS, in some key ways, is like that experienced by inmates of "total institutions" (e.g., mental asylums, prisons, the military). According to Goffman (1961: 16), the "inmate finds that certain roles are lost to him by virtue of the barrier that separates him from the outside world." In turn, there is an assault on the

self, or self-mortification. Through stages in a "moral career," a new social identity or self (e.g., mental patient, prisoner, solider) emerges based on interactions within the new constraints of institutional life.

I have used the phrase "social interaction" to highlight the work of Goffman and the phrase "social performances" to highlight that of Berger and Luckmann. Although these are different approaches with different key assumptions, both share the notion of a self as socially enacted. According to Berger and Luckmann, for example: "Both self and other can be apprehended as performers of objective, generally known actions, which are recurrent and repeatable by any actor of the appropriate type." Moreover, they continue, "The self is objectified *as* the performer" of actions (Berger and Luckmann 1967: 72, 73).

Chapter 4

1. Wendy's description of the cumulative impact of FMS as a "domino effect" is shared by Kathleen Kerry (2002) in her recent memoir about living with FMS, *Dominoes.*

2. For a general theoretical discussion of the mortification of self, see Goffman (1961).

3. The idea that FMS is a metaphorical bowl of marbles is also found in Bruce Campbell's (2003) online book found on a popular Web site (http://www.cfidsselfhelp.org). The "bowl of marbles" seems to be a popular and compelling metaphor for FMS; two other women in this study mentioned it during the course of their interview. Parenthetically, Campbell's description of an "energy bank account" closely parallels the economy of the body: "Think of yourself as having an energy bank account which has a very low balance." He continues the analogy noting there are "overdraws" and "service charges" if inadequate "deposits" are made.

4. One can plausibly claim that being unaware of the body in states of health is more taken-for-granted by men than women. It is the case that dramatic bodily changes are a regular part of women's lives (e.g., menstruation, pregnancy, menopause). It is important to note, however, that these dramatic changes do not signify ill health. For example, pregnancy is a normal aspect of women's embodiment and, even as the body appears anew, it does not appear as problematic (Young 1990). In addition, standards of youth and beauty make women more aware of their "normal" body and more committed to its alteration than are men. Therefore, although I acknowledge critiques that the phenomenological claim of the taken-for-granted body has a male bias in these particular ways, this does not undermine the argument here. The taken-for-granted ability (indeed, necessity) to organize everyday life "around the 'here' of my body," to return to Berger and Luckmann's language, is a phenomenological starting point shared by all members of society. The body's ability to move women through the routine of daily life is not severed in response to these female experiences, although it may be temporarily disrupted in response to pregnancy or childbirth—at least biologically, although it maybe culturally (e.g., menstrual taboos). In contrast, the

symptoms of FMS do represent a profound barrier to routine bodily movement and sever the sufferer from the world that is routinely under her bodily manipulation. Moreover, the symptoms present themselves as problematic and in sharp contrast to the pre-FMS body. In other words, what is taken for granted is not a complete lack of consciousness about the body, but a lack of consciousness about the routine body that makes actions and interactions physically possible.

Chapter 5

1. Almost every woman asked if I believed FMS was "real" before she agreed to an interview. I approached the question with trepidation. I neither wanted to misrepresent myself nor bias my sample by answering in a way that systematically encouraged some sufferers to participate while systematically discouraging others. My solution was to respond as a sociologist. I started by explicitly stating the cultural assumptions embedded in the question itself: "You mean, do I believe FMS is a disease with an organic cause?" From here, it was easy for me to answer truthfully that biomedical researchers would ultimately determine the answer to that question. As a sociologist, I assured them, I was more interested in, and more qualified to examine, what we culturally define as "real" and the concrete implications of that definition in terms of their experience. My honesty worked because it circumvented a tension that an FMS sufferer negotiates, namely the friction between her personal certainty and persistent public doubt about the legitimacy of her symptoms.

2. Although the percentage of women in medicine has been steadily rising since the 1970s, women physicians are still significantly underrepresented. According to the American Medical Association (2004), 25 percent of all physicians in 2002 (excluding students) were women.

3. In addition to demanding women's active role in their own medical decision-making, the feminist women's health movement also demanded a deprofessionalization of medical services and the demedicalization of women's health. The legalization of lay midwifery, for example, was a key demand of the movement, as were demands to restrict medicine's authority over women's bodies by encouraging women to care for their own health, as widely promoted in the popular self-help book, *Our Bodies, Ourselves*. These more radical impulses have not become culturally institutionalized, in large measure, because the spirit of the women's health movement has been co-opted by profit-oriented medical care providers. Women's health services are now big business and the medical provider industry sells "women-centered" health services, sans the radical impulses, fully entrenched within orthodox medical control (Satel 2000).

Chapter 6

1. In the few cases where such details were not volunteered, the women were directly asked to talk about how their condition was diagnosed, who diagnosed it, and how hearing the diagnosis made them feel.

2. Rheumatologists diagnosed the condition of eighteen of the twenty-six women who participated in the in-depth interviews. Three women learned of their diagnosis from other specialists (a neurologist, an orthopedic surgeon, and a physician in a pain and spine clinic); the remaining five were diagnosed by their general practitioner. Sixteen had never heard of FMS at the time of diagnosis; ten had heard of the diagnosis in advance; and, of these, four "actively" pursued an FMS diagnosis based on that information. The four women who participated only in the focus group interview were not asked questions about their diagnosing practitioner. Interestingly, none of men in this study were diagnosed by a rheumatologist. Two received their diagnosis from internists, one from a neurologists, and one from a psychiatrist.

3. Three women had their condition diagnosed before the ACR criteria were formalized, all three by rheumatologists. Recall from Chapter 1, rheumatologists used tender points to diagnose fibrositis or fibromyalgia well in advance of the ACR criteria.

4. Seven of the women were covered by the state's health program and the rest were insured through private health maintenance organizations (HMOs) or preferred provider organizations (PPOs).

5. An even more pronounced discrepancy appears between the first onset of FMS symptoms to diagnosis. For women, the average number of years is a just slightly more than thirteen; for men, the average is eighteen and a half.

Chapter 7

1. An earlier version of this chapter appears in *Social Problems*, 2002, Vol. 49, No. 3, pp. 279–300. In the article version, a quote from Wendy was incorrectly attributed to Alice (Barker 2002: 291). This quote now is correctly attributed to Wendy (see page 158). Five additional interviews were conducted after the article's publication. A final discrepancy: Pamela, who was quoted once in the article version, is referred to as Joyce throughout this book.

2. For an excellent review of the identity formation literature see Cerulo (1997).

3. Elaine Showalter (1997) makes such an argument in her book *Hystories: Hysterical Epidemics and Modern Media.*

4. Once the FMS sufferer finds her way to any of the several hundred FMS Web sites, for example, the provided links to the FMS community make possible a long journey, navigating from site to site in what appears to be a never-ending procession. Eventually, however, the procession returns to several sites over and again—sites that are linked to nearly all the others. Even while the FMS self-help and support community is bounded virtually, the community is by no means exclusively virtual. For example, on several FMS Web sites the visitor can find the date, time, and location of a real support group in her hometown and begin attending the group's regular sessions.

5. Thomasina Borkman (1999) provides a persuasive justification for using the terms "mutual aid" and "mutual help" rather than "self-help" in order to capture

the collective nature of these endeavors. Borkman (1999: 4–5) uses these terms to "refer to cases of reciprocal assistance whether or not self-help is present." This is a useful and clarifying point. Yet, in the process of making her argument, she defines support groups as "professionally managed groups of people who have the same problem" (Borkman 1999: 4). Although Borkman's attempt to sort out the important conceptual distinctions at play is a worthwhile enterprise, the term "support group" is widely used by the lay public to describe mutual aid and mutual help groups, including those free of professional oversight. In fact, in the FMS community, it is the preferred term used by lay groups to describe (and name) their own mutual aid/mutual help groups. Therefore, the term "support group" will be used in this study to describe all mutual aid/mutual help groups, whether or not they are professionally affiliated or autonomous.

6. Since the analysis for this chapter was completed, dozens of new FMS books have come on the market and some of them have become very popular. As noted, *A Survival Manual* remains the best selling book and the highest ranked by distribution demand (as of January 2003). The remaining four books, however, have been bumped from the top-five highest in demand. As of January 2003, distribution rankings for these four books were as follows: Elrod (sixth); Fransen and Russell (tenth); Williamson (fourteenth), and McIlwain and Bruce (twentieth). The top five books in terms of distribution demand as of January 2003, were: (1) Devin Starlanyl (2001), *Fibromyalgia and Chronic Myofascial Pain: A Survival Manual;* (2) Mark Pellegrino (2001), *Inside Fibromyalgia with Mark J. Pellegrino, M.D.: The New Prescription for Healing;* (3) Paul St. Amand (1999), *What Your Doctor May Not Tell You About Fibromyalgia: The Revolutionary Treatment That Can Reverse the Disease;* (4) Julie Kelly (1998), *Taking Charge of Fibromyalgia: A Self-Management Program for Your Fibromyalgia Syndrome;* and (5) Chet Cunningham (2000), *The Fibromyalgia Relief Handbook.* The changes in distribution demand from 2000 to 2003 are to be expected, given that, as a general rule, newer books tend to be in higher demand. The analysis presented here is based on the most popular books as of January 2000, knowing that these books had already influenced those living with fibromyalgia, including the women interviewed in this study in 2000–01.

7. Although not the empirical approach used in this chapter, one can also see parallels between the stories told by the interviewees and the narratives presented in best-selling books. Relating experiences within the cyclical framework of intense "flares" brought on by "triggers" is an obvious case in point. For example, the following description of flares in *A Survival Manual* closely parallels two of the women's accounts. "Flares are usually triggered by one or more activities or stressors. It might be something microscopically small, such as a virus . . . or something large and dramatic, such as a traffic accident" (Starlanyl and Copeland 1996: 127). From Sally: "It was my first flare. I don't know what caused it. It was such a long time ago, but it can be anything like the flu or a injury, like from a car accident." From Suzanne: "Sometimes it doesn't take anything real big and sometimes it is something big and traumatic, a car accident or different things." In many similar examples, women are clearly appropriating the narrative framework presented in the self-help books to organize their own FMS story.

8. All of these daily annoyances are cited as potential FMS symptoms in *A Survival Manual*. For example, tripping, spilling food and drinks, blotchy skins and illegible handwriting, and transposing letters and numbers (Starlanyl and Copeland 1996: 98, 157, 70, 85, and 171).

9. This findings is consistent with other research indicating an average of five to seven years of acute symptoms prior to be diagnosed with FMS (Goldenberg 1999).

10. The lobbying efforts of Fibromyalgia Network also led to the first federal National Institutes of Health monies available for FMS research in 1999.

Chapter 8

1. This study did not use the ACR criteria to diagnose FMS.

2. Most research into the differential effects of education explores its effects on income, occupation, and prestige. In other words, researchers have illustrated that the ability to trade in on educational investments differs not only by class, but also by race and gender (Anderson and Shapiro 1996; Ashraf 1994; Monk-Turner 1994). It follows from this research that education's effect on health outcomes would differ according to class, gender, and race status.

3. One of the most important social scientific works in the area of MCS makes no mention of the racial composition of their research subjects (Kroll-Smith and Floyd 1997).

4. By drawing attention to a *normalization* of suffering among black women relative to white women, it is not my intent to reproduce destructive imagery that has been used to reinforce racial equality. It is not my intent, for instance, to suggest that the strong black "matriarch" is somehow responsible for her own failure, the failure of her children, and the failure of the black community (Collins 1991).

Bibliography/Works Cited

Abbey, Susan and Paul E. Garfinkel. 1991. "Neurasthenia and chronic fatigue syndrome: The role of culture in the making of a diagnosis." *American Journal of Psychiatry* 148: 1638–46.

Abbott, Andrew. 1988. *The System of Professions: An Essay on the Division of Expert Labor.* Chicago: University of Chicago Press.

Abeles, Micha. 1998. "Fibromyalgia syndrome." Pp. 32–57 in *Functional Somatic Syndromes: Etiology, Diagnosis, and Treatment,* edited by P. Manu. Cambridge, England: Cambridge University Press.

Adisa, Opal Palmer. 1990. "Rocking in the sun light: Stress and black women." Pp. 11–14 in *The Black Women's Health Book,* edited by E. C. White. Seattle: Seal Press.

American Board of Internal Medicine. 2004. "Number of diplomates." Retrieved July 29, 2004 (http://www.abim.org/resources/dnum.shtm).

American Medical Association. 2004. "Physicians by gender." Retrieved July 28, 2004, 2004 (http://www.ama-assn.org/ama/pub/article/171–195.html).

American Psychiatric Association. 1980. *Diagnostic and Statistical Manual of Mental Disorders.* Washington, DC

Amir, M., Z. Kaplan, L. Neumann, R. Sharabani, N. Shani, and D. Buskila. 1997. "Post-traumatic stress disorder, tenderness and fibromyalgia." *Journal of Psychosomatic Research* 42: 607–13.

Anderberg, U.M., Z. Liu, L. Berglund, and F. Nyberg. 1998. "Plasma levels on nociception in female fibromyalgia syndrome patients." *Zeitschrift fur Rheumatologie* 57: 77–80.

Anderson, Deborah and David Shapiro. 1996. "Racial differences in access to high-paying jobs and the wage gap between black and white women." *Industrial and Labor Relations Review* 49: 273–86.

Anson, O., S. Carmel, and M. Levin. 1991. "Gender differences in the utilization of emergency department services." *Women and Health* 17: 91–104.

Aronowitz, Robert. 1998. *Making Sense of Illness: Science, Society, and Disease.* Cambridge: Cambridge University Press.

Arthritis Foundation. 2003. "Speaking of pain: How to talk with your doctor about pain." Retrieved June 20, 2003 (http://www.arthritis.org/conditions/speakingofpain/).

Asbring, Pia and Anna-Liisa Narvanen. 2003. "Ideal versus reality: Physicians' perspectives on patients with chronic fatigue syndrome (CFS) and fibromyalgia." *Social Science and Medicine* 57: 711–20.

Ashraf, Javed. 1994. "Differences in returns to education: An analysis by race." *American Journal of Economics and Sociology* 53: 281–90.

Baldwin, C.M., I.R. Bell, M. Fernandez, and G.E.R. Schwartz. 2000. "Multiple chemical sensitivity." Pp. 1110–19 in *Women and Health*, edited by M. B. Goldman and M. C. Hatch. New York: Academic Press.

Banks, Jonathan and Lindsay Prior. 2001. "Doing things with illness: The micro politics of the CFS clinic." *Social Science and Medicine* 52: 11–23.

Barker, Kristin. 2002. "The making of fibromyalgia syndrome." *Social Problems* 49: 279–300.

Barsky, Arthur and Jonathan Borus. 1995. "Somatization and medicalization in the era of managed care." *JAMA* 274: 1931–34.

———. 1999. "Functional somatic syndromes." *Annals of Internal Medicine* 130: 910–21.

Bartley, M., J. Popay, and J. Plewis. 1992. "Domestic conditions, paid employment and women's experiences of ill health." *Sociology of Health and Illness* 14: 313–41.

Baszanger, Isabelle. 1995. *Inventing Pain Medicine: From Laboratory to the Clinic.* New Brunswick, NJ: Rutgers University Press.

Bennett, Robert. 1999a. "A contemporary overview of fibromyalgia." National Fibromyalgia Research Foundation Conference. Portland, Oregon, September 26–27.

———. 1999b. "Emerging concepts in the neurobiology of chronic pain: Evidence of abnormal sensory processing in fibromyalgia." *Mayo Clinic Proc* 74: 385–98.

———. 2003. "The scientific basis for understanding pain in fibromyalgia." Oregon Fibromyalgia Foundation. Retrieved January 6, 2003 (http://www.myalgia.com).

Berger, Peter and Thomas Luckmann. 1967. *The Social Construction of Reality: A Treatise in the Sociology of Knowledge.* New York: Anchor.

Berkley, Karen. 1992. "Vive la difference." *Trends Neuroscience* 15: 331–32.

Berman, B.M. and J.P. Swyers. 1999. "Complementary medicine treatments for fibromyalgia syndrome." *Bailliere's Best Practice and Research in Clinical Rheumatology* 13: 487–92.

Bill-Harvey, D., R.M. Rippey, M. Abeles, and C.A. Pfeiffer. 1989. "Methods used by urban, low-income minorities to care for their arthritis." *Arthritis Care and Research* 2: 60–64.

Bird, Chloe and Patricia Rieker. 1999. "'Gender matters': An integrated model for understanding men's and women's health." *Social Science and Medicine* 48: 745–55.

Block, Sidney. 1999. "On the nature of rheumatism." *Arthritis and Rheumatism* 12: 129–38.

Bohr, T. 1995. "Fibromyalgia syndrome and myofascial pain syndrome. Do they exist?" *Neurologic Clinics* 13: 365–84.

———. 1996. "Problems with myofascial pain syndrome and fibromyalgia syndrome." *Neurology* 46: 593–97.

Boisset-Pioro, M.H., J.M. Esdaile, and M.A. Fitzcharles. 1995. "Sexual and physical abuse in women with fibromyalgia syndrome." *Arthritis and Rheumatism* 38: 235–41.

Boland, E.W. 1947. "Psychogenic rheumatism: The musculoskeletal expression of psychoneurosis." *Annals of Rheumatic Disease* 6: 195.

Borkman, Thomasina. 1999. *Understanding Self-Help/Mutual Aid: Experiential Learning in the Commons.* New Brunswick, NJ: Rutgers University Press.

Boulware, L.E., L.A. Cooper, L.E. Ratner, T.A. LaVeist, and N.R. Powe. 2003. "Race and trust in the health care system." *Public Health Reports* 118: 358–65.

Bourdieu, Pierre. 1984. *Distinctions: A Social Critique of Judgment and Taste.* Cambridge, MA: Harvard University Press.

Bourdieu, Pierre and Loic J.D. Wacquant. 1992. *An Invitation to Reflexive Sociology.* Chicago: University of Chicago Press.

Broom, Dorothy and Roslyn Woodward. 1996. "Medicalisation reconsidered: Toward a collaborative approach to care." *Sociology of Health and Illness* 18: 357–78.

Brown, Phil. 1995. "Naming and framing: The social construction of diagnosis and illness." *Journal of Health and Social Behavior* 34–52.

Brumberg, Joan. 1992. "From psychiatric syndrome to 'communicable' disease: The case of anorexia nervosa." Pp. 134–54 in *Framing Disease: Studies in Cultural History,* edited by C. Rosenberg and J. Golden. New Brunswick, NJ: Rutgers University Press.

Burckhardt, C.S., S.R. Clark, and R.M. Bennett. 1993. "Fibromyalgia and quality of life: A comparative analysis." *Journal of Rheumatology* 20: 275–79.

Bury, Michael. 1982. "Chronic illness as biographical disruption." *Sociology of Health and Illness* 4: 167–82.

Buskila, D., L. Neumann, A. Alhoashle, and M. Abu-Shakra. 2000. "Fibromyalgia syndrome in men." *Seminars in Arthritis and Rheumatism* 30: 47–51.

Buskila, D., L. Neumann, I. Hazanov, and R. Carmi. 1996. "Familial aggregation in the fibromyalgia syndrome." *Seminars in Arthritis and Rheumatism* 26: 605–11.

Byrd, W. Michael and Linda A. Clayton. 2000–2002. *An American Health Dilemma: Race, Medicine and Health Care in the United States, 1900–2000.* New York: Routledge.

Cain, Carole. 1991. "Personal stories: Identity acquisition and self-understanding in Alcoholics Anonymous." *Ethos* 19: 210–53.

Calderone, Karen. 1990. "The influence of gender on the frequency of pain and sedative medication administered to postoperative patients." *Sex Roles* 23: 713–25.

Campbell, Bruce. 2003. *The CFIDS and Fibromyalgia Self-Help Book.* Retrieved May 15, 2004 (http://www.cfidsselfhelp.org/).

Carrette, S. 1995. "What have clinical trails taught us about the treatment of fibromyalgia?" *Journal of Musculoskeletal Pain* 3: 133–49.

Cerulo, Karen. 1997. "Identity construction: New issues, new directions." *Annual Review of Sociology* 23: 385–409.

Charmaz, Kathy. 1991. *Good Days, Bad Days: The Self in Chronic Illness and Time.* New Brunswick, NJ: Rutgers University Press.

Chodorow, Nancy. 1978. *The Reproduction of Mothering: Psychoanalysis and the Sociology of Gender.* Berkeley, CA: University of California Press.

Clarke, Adele and Virginia Olesen. 1999. *Revisioning Women, Health, and Healing.* New York: Routledge.

Clarke, Adele, Laura Mamo, Jennifer R. Fishman, Janet K. Shim, and Jennifer Ruth Fosket. 2003. "Biomedicalization: Technoscientific transformations of health, illness, and U.S. biomedicine." *American Sociological Review* 68: 161–94.

Clements, A., M. Sharpe, S. Simkin, J. Borrill, and K. Hawton. 1997. "Chronic fatigue syndrome: A qualitative investigation of patients' beliefs about the illness." *Journal of Psychosomatic Research* 42: 615–24.

Cognitive Science Laboratory. 2005. "Wordnet." Princeton University. Retrieved January 29, 2005 (http://wordnet.princeton.edu).

Cohen, H., L. Neumann, Y. Haiman, M.A. Matar, J. Press, and D. Buskila. 2002. "Prevalence of post-traumatic stress disorder in fibromyalgia patients: Overlapping syndromes or post-traumatic fibromyalgia syndrome?" *Seminars in Arthritis and Rheumatism* 32: 38–50.

Cohen, Milton. 1999. "Is fibromyalgia a distinct clinical entity? The disapproving rheumatologist's evidence." *Bailliere's Clinical Rheumatology* 12: 421–25.

Collins, Patricia Hill. 1991. *Black Feminist Thought: Knowledge, Consciousness, and the Politics of Empowerment.* New York: Routledge.

Conrad, Peter. 1987. "The experience of illness: Recent and new directions." *Research in the Sociology of Health Care* 6: 1–31.

Conrad, Peter and Deborah Potter. 2000. "From hyperactive children to ADHD adults: Observations on the expansion of medical categories." *Social Problems* 47: 559–82.

Conrad, Peter and Joseph W. Schneider. 1992. *Deviance and Medicalization: From Badness to Sickness.* Philadelphia: Temple University Press.

Cooper, Lesley. 1997. "Myalgic encephalomyelitis and the medical encounter." *Sociology of Health and Illness* 19: 186–207.

Crofford, Leslie and B.E. Appleton. 2001. "Complementary and alternative therapies for fibromyalgia." *Current Rheumatology Reports* 3: 147–56.

Crofford, Leslie and Daniel Clauw. 2002. "Fibromyalgia: Where are we a decade after the American College of Rheumatology classification criteria were developed?" *Arthritis and Rheumatism* 46: 1136–38.

Crofford, Leslie, N.C. Engleberg, and M. Demitrack. 1996. "Neurohormonal perturbations in fibromyalgia." *Bailliere's Clinical Rheumatology* 10: 365–78.

Croft, Peter and Alan J. Silman. 1999. Introduction. *Bailliere's Clinical Rheumatology* 13: ix–xii.

Csillag, Claudio. 1992. "Fibromyalgia: The Copenhagen declaration." *Lancet* 340: 663–64.

da Silva, Luiz Claudio. 2004. "Fibromyalgia. Reflections about empirical science and faith." *Journal of Rheumatology* 31: 827–28.

Davis, Angela Y. 1990. "Sick and tired of being sick and tired: The politics of black women's health." Pp. 18–26 in *The Black Women's Health Book*, edited by E. C. White. Seattle: Seal Press.

Davis, Bridgett M. 1990. "Speaking of grief: Today I feel real low, I hope you understand." Pp. 219–225 in *The Black Women's Health Book*, edited by E. C. White. Seattle: Seal Press.

Davis, Kathy. 1988. *Power Under the Microscope*. Providence, RI: Foris.

de Beauvoir, Simone. 1989 [1953]. *The Second Sex*. Translated by H. M. Parshley. New York: Knopf.

de Swaan, A. 1989. "The reluctant imperialism of the medical profession." *Social Science and Medicine* 28: 1165–70.

Descartes, René. 1951 [1641]. *Meditations*. Translated by L. J. Lafleur. New York: Liberal Arts Press.

Didi-Huberman, Georges. 2003. *Invention of Hysteria: Charcot and the Photographic Iconography of the Salpêtrière*. Translated by A. Hartz. Cambridge, MA: MIT Press.

Doyal, Lesley. 1995. *What Makes Women Sick: Gender and the Political Economy of Health*. New Brunswick, NJ: Rutgers University Press.

Durkheim, Emile. 1964 [1893]. *The Division of Labor in Society*. Translated by G. Simpson. New York: Free Press.

———. 1995 [1912]. *The Elementary Forms of Religious Life*. Translated by K. E. Fields. New York: Free Press.

Ehrenreich, Barbara and Deirdre English. 1973. *Complaints and Disorders: The Sexual Politics of Sickness*. New York: Feminist Press.

Ehrlich, George E. 2003a. "Fibromyalgia is not a diagnosis: Comment on the editorial by Crofford and Clauw." *Arthritis and Rheumatism* 48: 276.

———. 2003b. "Pain is real; Fibromyalgia isn't." *Journal of Rheumatology* 30: 1666.

Ellis, R.P. 1998. "Creaming, skimping and dumping: Provider competition on the intensive and extensive margins." *Journal of Health Economics* 17: 537–55.

Elrod, Joe. 1997. *Reversing Fibromyalgia*. Pleasant Grove, UT: Woodland Publishing.

Emanuel, E.J. and N.N. Dubler. 1995. "Preserving the physician-patient relationship in the era of managed care." *JAMA* 273: 323–29.

Estroff, Sue E., William S. Lachicotte, Linda C. Illingworth, and Anna Johnson. 1991. "Everybody's got a little mental illness: Accounts of illness and self among people with severe, persistent mental illness." *Medical Anthropology Quarterly* 5: 331–69.

Ezzy, Douglas. 2000. "Illness narratives: Time, hope and HIV." *Social Science and Medicine* 50: 605–17.

Faucett, Julia. 1997. "The ergonomics of women's work." Pp. 154–72 in *Women's Health: Complexities and Differences*, edited by S. B. Ruzek, V. Olsen, and A. Clarke. Columbus, OH: Ohio State University Press.

Fillingim, Roger. 2000. *Sex, Gender, and Pain.* Seattle: IASP Press.

Finkler, Kaja. 1994. *Women in Pain: Gender and Morbidity in Mexico.* Philadelphia: University of Pennsylvania Press.

Foucault, Michel. 1975. *The Birth of the Clinic: An Archaeology of Medical Perception.* New York: Vintage.

———. 1977. *Discipline and Punish: The Birth of the Prison.* New York: Vintage.

Frank, Arthur. 1991. *At the Will of the Body: Reflections on Illness.* Boston: Houghton Mifflin.

———. 1995. *The Wounded Storyteller: Body, Illness, and Ethics.* Chicago: University of Chicago Press.

Franke, Nikki V. 1997. "African American women's health: The effects of disease and chronic life stressors." Pp. 353–79 in *Women's Health: Complexities and Differences,* edited by S. B. Ruzek, V. Olsen, and A. Clarke. Columbus, OH: Ohio State University Press.

Frankenhaeuser, Frank, Ulf Lundberg, and Margaret Chesney. 1991. *Women, Work, and Health: Stress and Opportunities.* New York: Plenum Press.

Fransen, Jenny and I. Jon. Russell. 1996. *The Fibromyalgia Help Book: Practical Guide to Living Better with Fibromyalgia.* St. Paul, MN: Smith House Press.

Freidson, Eliot. 1971. *Profession of Medicine: A Study of the Sociology of Applied Knowledge.* New York: Harper and Row.

Freund, Peter E.S., Meredith B. McGuire, and Linda S. Podhurst. 2003. *Health, Illness, and the Social Body: A Critical Sociology.* Upper Saddle River, NJ: Prentice Hall.

Friedan, Betty. 1963. *The Feminine Mystique.* New York: Norton.

Friedman, A.W., M.B. Tewi, C. Ahn, G. Jr. McGwin, B.J. Fessler, H.M. Bastian, B.A. Baethge, J.D. Reveille, and G.S. Alarcon. 2003. "Systemic lupus erythematosus in three ethnic groups: XV. Prevalence and correlates of fibromyalgia." *Lupus* 12: 274–79.

Garro, Linda. 1994. "Narrative representations of chronic illness experience: Cultural models of illness, mind and body in stories concerning the temporomandibular joint (TMJ)." *Social Science and Medicine* 38: 775–88.

Geronimus, A.T. 2001. "Understanding and eliminating racial inequalities in women's health in the United States: The role of weathering conceptual framework." *Journal of the American Medical Women's Association* 56: 133–36, 149–50.

Giddens, Anthony. 1991. *Modernity and Self-Identity: Self and Society in the Late Modern Age.* Stanford, CA: Stanford University Press.

Gilligan, Carol. 1982. *In a Different Voice: Psychological Theory and Women's Development.* Cambridge, MA: Harvard University Press.

Gillum, R.F. 1996. "Epidemiology of hypertension in African American women." *American Heart Journal* 131: 385–95.

Goetz, Christopher G., Michel Bonduelle, and Toby Gelfand. 1995. *Charcot: Constructing Neurology.* New York: Oxford University Press.

Goffman, Erving. 1961. *Asylums: Essays on the Social Situation of Mental Patients and Other Inmates.* Garden City, NJ: Doubleday.

Goldenberg, Don. 1999. "Fibromyalgia syndrome a decade later: What have we learned?" *Archives of Internal Medicine* 159: 777–85.

———. 2002. "Office management of fibromyalgia." *Rheumatic Disease Clinics of North America* 28: 437–46.

Goldenberg, Don, Carole Burckhardt, and Leslie Crofford. 2004. "Management of fibromyalgia syndrome." *JAMA* 292: 2388–95.

Goldenberg, Don, C.J. Mossey, and C.H. Schmid. 1995. "A model to assess severity and impact of fibromyalgia." *Journal of Rheumatology* 22: 2313–18.

Goldenberg, Don and Nicole Smith. 2003. "Fibromyalgia, rheumatologists, and the medical literature: A shaky alliance." *Journal of Rheumatology* 30: 151–53.

Good, Byron J. 1994. *Medicine, Rationality, and Experience: An Anthropological Perspective.* New York: Cambridge University Press.

Good, Mary-Jo DelVecchio, Paul E. Brodwin, Byron J. Good, and Arthur Kleinman. 1992. *Pain as Human Experience: An Anthropological Perspective.* Berkeley, CA: University of California Press.

Graham, Hilary. 1993. *Hardship and Health in Women's Lives.* New York: Harvester Wheatsheaf.

Gran, Jan Tore. 2003. "The epidemiology of chronic generalized musculoskeletal pain." *Best Practices and Research Clinical Rheumatology* 17: 547–61.

Greenhalgh, Susan. 2001. *Under the Medical Gaze: Facts and Fictions of Chronic Pain.* Berkeley, CA: University of California Press.

Hacking, Ian. 1999. *The Social Construction of What?* Cambridge, MA: Harvard University Press.

Hadler, N.M. 1996. "If you have to prove you are ill, you can't get well. The object lesson of fibromyalgia." *Spine* 21: 2397–400.

———. 1997a. "Fibromyalgia, chronic fatigue, and other iatrogenic diagnostic algorithms. Do some labels escalate illness in vulnerable patients?" *Postgraduate Medicine* 102: 262–77.

———. 1997b. "La maladie est morte, vive le malade (The disease is dead, long live the disease)." *Journal of Rheumatology* 24: 1250–51.

———. 1999. "Fibromyalgia: Could it Be In Your Mind?" Rheuma21st. Retrieved February 15, 2001 (http://www.rheuma21st.com/archives/cutting_edge_fibromyalgia.html).

Hallberg, Lillemore R.M. and Sven G. Carlsson. 1998. "Psychosocial vulnerability and maintaining forces related to fibromyalgia." *Scandinavian Journal of Caring Sciences* 12: 95–103.

Hamelsky, Sanda W., Walter F. Stewart, and Richard B. Lipton. 2000. "Epidemiology of headache in women: Emphasis on migraine." Pp. 1084–97 in *Women and Health,* edited by M. B. Goldman and M. C. Hatch. New York: Academic Press.

Harris-Lacewell, Melissa. 2001. "No place to rest: African American political attitudes and the myth of black women's strength." *Women and Politics* 23: 1–33.

Hawley, Donna and Frederick Wolfe. 2000. "Fibromyalgia." Pp. 1068–83 in *Women and Health,* edited by M. B. Goldman and M. C. Hatch. New York: Academic Press.

Hayden, Lars-Christer and Lisbeth Sacks. 1998. "Suffering, hope and diagnosis: On negotiation of chronic fatigue syndrome." *Health* 2: 175–93.

Hays, Sharon. 2003. *Flat Broke with Children: Women in the Age of Welfare Reform.* New York: Oxford University Press.

Hellström, Olle, J. Bullington, G. Karlsson, P. Lindqvist P, and B. Mattsson. 1998. "Doctors' attitudes to fibromyalgia: A phenomenological study." *Scandinavian Journal of Social Medicine* 26: 232–37.

————. 1999. "A phenomenological study of fibromyalgia: Patient perspectives." *Scandinavian Journal of Primary Health Care* 17: 11–16.

Henriksson, C. and C. Burckhardt. 1996. "Impact of fibromyalgia on everyday life: A study of women in the USA and Sweden." *Disability and Rehabilitation* 18: 241–48.

Henriksson, Karl. 2002. "Is fibromyalgia a central pain state?" *Journal of Musculoskeletal Pain* 10: 45–57.

Hibbard, Judith and Clyde Pope. 1983. "Gender roles, illness orientation and use of medical services." *Social Science and Medicine* 17: 129–37.

————. 1986. "Another look at sex differences in the use of medical care: Illness orientation and the types of morbidities in which services are used." *Women and Health* 11: 21–36.

Hilbert, Richard. 1984. "The acultural dimensions of chronic pain: Flawed reality construction and the problem of meaning." *Social Problems* 31: 365–78.

Hochschild, Arlie. 1983. *The Managed Heart: The Commercialization of Human Feelings.* Berkeley, CA: University of California Press.

————. 1990. *The Second Shift.* New York: Avon.

Hoffmann, D.E. and A.J. Tarzian. 2001. "The girl who cried pain: A bias against women in the treatment of pain." *The Journal of Law, Medicine and Ethics* 29: 13–27.

Hooks, Bell. 1984. *Feminist Theory from Margin to Center.* Boston: South End Press.

Hudson, J.I. and H.G. Jr. Pope. 1989. "Fibromyalgia and psychopathology: Is fibromyalgia a form of 'affective spectrum disorder?' " *Journal of Rheumatology* 19: 15–22.

————. 1996. "The relationship between fibromyalgia and major depressive disorder." *Rheumatic Disease Clinics of North America* 22: 285–303.

Illich, Ivan. 1976. *Medical Nemesis: The Expropriation of Health.* New York: Pantheon.

Irvine, Leslie. 1999. *Codependent Forevermore: The Invention of Self in a Twelve Step Group.* Chicago: University of Chicago Press.

Jacobsson, L.T., D.K. Nagi, S.R. Pillemer, W.C. Knowler, R.L. Hanson, D.J. Pettitt, and P.H. Bennett. 1996. "Low prevalences of chronic widespread pair and shoulder disorders among Pima Indians." *Journal of Rheumatology* 23: 907–09.

Kalben, Barbara Blatt. 2003. "Why men die younger: Causes of mortality differences in sex." Society of Actuaries. Retrieved July 18, 2003 (http://www.soa.org).

Kaminer, Wendy. 1999. *Sleeping with Extra-Terrestrials.* New York: Vintage.

Kaplan, Jonathan Michael. 2000. *The Limits and Lies of Human Genetic Research: Dangers for Social Policy.* New York: Routledge.

Kerry, Kathleen. 2002. *Dominoes: A Memoir.* Lynnwood, WA: Lemonade Press.

Kersley, George and John Glyn. 1991. *A Concise International History of Rheumatology and Rehabilitation: Friends and Foes.* New York: The Royal Society of Medicine Services Limited.

Kleinman, Arthur. 1986. *Social Origins of Distress and Disease: Neurasthenia, Depression, and Pain in Modern China.* New Haven, CT: Yale University Press.

———. 1988. *The Illness Narratives: Suffering, Healing and the Human Condition.* New York: Basic Books.

Korszun, A., E.A. Young, N.C. Engleberg, L. Masterson, E.C. Dawson, K. Spindler, L.A. McClure, M.B. Brown, and L.J. Crofford. 2000. "Follicular phase hypothalamic-pituitary-gonadal axis function in women with fibromyalgia and chronic fatigue syndrome." *The Journal of Rheumatology* 27: 1526–30.

Kroll-Smith, Steve and Hugh H. Floyd. 1997. *Bodies in Protest: Environmental Illness and the Struggle over Medical Knowledge.* New York: New York University Press.

Kugelmann, Robert. 1999. "Complaining about chronic pain." *Social Science and Medicine* 49: 1663–76.

Lamont, Michele. 1992. *Money, Morals, and Manners: The Culture of the French and the American Upper Middle Class.* Chicago: University of Chicago Press.

Laqueur, Thomas Walter. 1990. *Making Sex: Body and Gender from the Greeks to Freud.* Cambridge, MA: Harvard University Press.

Larson, M.S. 1977. *The Rise of Professionalism.* Berkeley, CA: University of California Press.

Leder, D. 1990. *The Absent Body.* Chicago: University of Chicago Press.

Ledingham, J., S. Doherty, and M. Doherty. 1993. "Primary fibromyalgia syndrome: An outcome study." *The British Journal of Rheumatology* 33: 139–42.

Legangneux, E., J.J. Mora, O. Spreux-Varoquaux, I. Thorin, M. Herrou, G. Alvado, and C. Gomeni. 2001. "Cerebrospinal fluid biogenic amine metabolites, plasma-rich platelet serotonin and [3H]imipramine reuptake in the primary fibromyalgia syndrome." *Rheumatology* 40: 290–96.

Lengermann, Patricia and Jill Niebrugge. 1995. "Intersubjectivity and domination: A feminist investigation of the sociology of Alfred Schutz." *Sociological Theory* 13: 25–36.

LeResche, Linda and Mark Drangsholt. 2000. "Temporomandibular disorder." Pp. 1120–28 in *Women and Health,* edited by M. B. Goldman and M. C. Hatch. New York: Academic Press.

Lorber, Judith. 1997. *Gender and the Social Construction of Illness.* Thousand Oaks, CA: Sage Publishing.

Makela, Matti Olli. 1999. "Is fibromyalgia a distinct clinical entity? The epidemiologist's evidence." *Bailliere's Clinical Rheumatology* 13: 415–19.

Makela, Matti Olli and M. Heliovaara. 1991. "Prevalence of primary fibromyalgia in the Finnish population." *British Medical Journal* 303: 216–19.

Mannheim, Karl. 1936. *Ideology and Utopia.* New York: Harcourt, Brace and Company.

Markens, Susan. 1996. "The problematic of 'experience': A political and cultural critique of PMS." *Gender and Society* 10: 42–58.

Martin, Emily. 1987. *The Woman in the Body: A Cultural Analysis of Reproduction.* Boston: Beacon Press, 1987.

————. 1991. "The egg and the sperm: How science has constructed a romance based on stereotypical male-female roles." *Signs* 16: 485–501.

Marx, Karl and Frederick Engels. 1973 [1932]. *The German Ideology.* New York: International Publishers.

Masi, Alfonse. 1998. "Concepts of illness in populations as applied to fibromyalgia syndromes: A biopsychosocial perspective." *Zeitschrift fur Rheumatologie* 57: 31–35.

Masi, Alfonse, K.P. White, and J.J. Pilcher. 2002. "Person-centered approach to care, teaching, and research in fibromyalgia syndrome: Justification from biopsychosocial perspective in populations." *Seminars in Arthritis and Rheumatism* 32: 71–93.

Matthews, Holly, Donald Lannin, and James Mitchell. 1994. "Coming to terms with advanced breast cancer: Black women's narratives from eastern North Carolina." *Social Science and Medicine* 38: 789–800.

McIlwain, Harris and Debra Fulghum Bruce. 1996. *The Fibromyalgia Handbook.* New York: Henry Holt.

McKinlay, John B. and Sonja M. McKinlay. 2001. "Medical measures and the decline of mortality." Pp. 7–19 in *The Sociology of Health and Illness: Critical Perspectives, 6th Edition,* edited by P. Conrad. New York: Worth Publishers.

Mead, Margaret. 1963 [1935]. *Sex and Temperament in Three Primitive Societies.* New York: W. Morrow and Company.

Mechanic, David. 1992. "Health and illness behavior and patient-practitioner relationships." *Social Science and Medicine* 34: 1345–50.

Melucci, Alberto. 1988. "Getting involved: Identity and mobilization in social movements." Pp. 329–48 in *From Structure to Action: Comparing Social Movement Research Across Cultures,* edited by B. Klandermans, K. Hanspeter, and S. Tarrow. Greenwich, CT: JAI Press.

Merton, Robert. 1973 [1945]. "Paradigm for the sociology of knowledge." Pp. 7–40 in *The Sociology of Science: Theory and Empirical Investigations,* edited by N. W. Storer. Chicago: Chicago University Press.

Micale, Mark S. 1995. *Approaching Hysteria: Disease and Its Interpretations.* Princeton, NJ: Princeton University Press.

Mills, C. Wright. 1959. *The Sociological Imagination.* New York: Oxford University Press.

Mink, Gwendolyn. 2002. *Welfare's End.* Ithaca, NY: Cornell University Press.

Mirowsky, John and Catherine E. Ross. 1995. "Sex differences in distress: Real or artificial?" *American Sociological Review* 60: 449–68.

Mishler, Elliot. 1984. *The Discourse of Medicine: Dialectics of Medical Interviews.* Norwood, New Jersey: Ablex Publishing Corporation.

Mitchell, Juliet. 1975. *Psychoanalysis and Feminism.* New York: Vintage Books.

Monk-Turner, Elizabeth. 1994. "Economic returns to community and four-year college education." *Journal of Socio-economics* 23: 441–47.

Morgan, M. 1996. "Prenatal care of African American women in selected USA urban and rural cultural contexts." *Journal of Transcultural Nursing* 7: 3–9.

Morgen, Sandra. 2002. *Into Our Own Hands: The Women's Health Movement in the United States, 1969–1990.* New Brunswick, NJ: Rutgers University Press.

Morris, David. 1991. *The Culture of Pain.* Berkeley, CA: University of California Press.

Mountz, J.M., L.A. Bradley, and G.S Alarcon. 1995. "Abnormal functional activity of the central nervous system in fibromyalgia syndrome." *American Journal of the Medical Sciences* 315: 385–96.

National Center for Health Statistics. 2000. *National Vital Statistics Report.* 48. Hyattsville, MD: National Center for Health Statistics.

———. 2001. "National Vital Statistics Reports, vol. 49, no. 12." National Center for Health Statistics. Retrieved June 19, 2004 (http://www.cdc.gov/nchs/data/nvsr/nvsr49/nvsr49_12.pdf).

Neumann, L. and D. Buskila. 1998. "Ethnocultural and educational differences in Israeli women correlate with pain perception in fibromyalgia." *Journal of Rheumatology* 25: 1369–73.

———. 2003. "Epidemiology of fibromyalgia." *Current Pain and Headache Reports* 7: 362–68.

Newman, Louise Michele. 1985. *Men's Ideas/Women's Realities: Popular Science, 1870–1915.* New York: Pergamon Press.

Oakley, Ann. 1993. *Essays on Women, Medicine and Health.* Edinburgh, Scotland: Edinburgh University Press.

Olsen, Virginia. 1997. "Who cares? Women as informal and formal caregivers." Pp. 397–424 in *Women's Health: Complexities and Differences,* edited by S. B. Ruzek, V. Olsen, and A. Clarke. Columbus, OH: Ohio State University Press.

Olson, James Stuart. 2002. *Bathsheba's Breast: Women, Cancer and History.* Baltimore: The Johns Hopkins University Press.

Ong, Aihwa. 1995. "Making the biopolitical subject: Cambodian immigrants, refugee medicine and cultural citizenship in California." *Social Science and Medicine* 40: 1243–57.

Ostensen, M., A. Rugelsjoen, and S.H. Wigers. 1997. "The effect of reproductive events and alterations of sex hormone levels on the symptoms of fibromyalgia." *Scandinavian Journal of Rheumatology.* 26: 355–60.

Osterweis, Marian, Arthur Kleinman, and David Mechanic, eds. 1987. *Pain and Disability: Clinical, Behavioral, and Public Policy Perspectives.* Washington, DC: National Academy Press.

Oudshoorn, Nelly. 1994. *Beyond The Natural Body: An Archeology of Sex Hormones.* New York: Routledge.

———. 1997. "Menopause, only for women? The social construction of menopause as an exclusively female condition." *Journal of Psychosomatic Obstetrics and Gynaecology* 18: 137–44.

Parsons, C. Lowell, Mehdi Kamarei, and Manoj Monga. 2000. "Interstitial cystitis." Pp. 1110–19 in *Women and Health,* edited by M. B. Goldman and M. C. Hatch. New York: Academic Press.

Parsons, Talcott. 1951. *The Social System.* Glencoe, IL: The Free Press.

Payne, T.C., F. Leavitt, D.C. Garron, R.S. Katz, H.E. Golden, P.B. Glickman, and C. Vanderplate. 1982. "Fibrositis and psychologic disturbance." *Arthritis and Rheumatism* 25: 213–17.

Peters, N., A. Rose, and K. Armstrong. 2004. "The association between race and attitudes about predictive genetic testing." *Cancer Epidemiology, Biomarkers and Prevention* 13: 361–65.

Phillips, Marilynn. 1990. "Damaged goods: Oral narratives of the experience of disability in American culture." *Social Science and Medicine* 30: 849–57.

Popay, J., M. Bartley, and C. Owne. 1993. "Gender inequalities in health: Social position, affective disorders and minor physical morbidity." *Social Science and Medicine* 36: 21–32.

Rafalovich, Adam. 1999. "Keep coming back! Narcotics Anonymous narrative and recovering-addict identity." *Contemporary Drug Problems* 26: 131–57.

Raphael, K.G. and J.J. Marbach. 2000. "Comorbid fibromyalgia accounts for reduced fecundity in women with myofascial face pain." *Clinical Journal of Pain* 16: 29–36.

Redondo, J.R., C.M. Justo, F.V. Moraleda, Y.G. Velayos, J.J. Puche, J.R. Zubero, T.G. Hernández, L.C. Ortells, and M.A. Pareja. 2004. "Long-term efficacy of therapy in patients with fibromyalgia: a physical exercise-based program and a cognitive-behavioral approach." *Arthritis and Rheumatism* 51: 184–92.

Reutter, L., A. Neufeld, and M.J. Harrison. 1998. "Nursing research on the health of low-income women." *Public Health Nursing* 15: 109–22.

Reynolds, M.D. 1983. "The development of the concept of fibrositis." *Journal of the History of Medicine and Allied Sciences* 38: 5–35.

Richman, Judith A. and Leonard A. Jason. 2001. "Gender biases underlying the social construction of illness states: The case of chronic fatigue syndrome." *Current Sociology* 49: 15–29.

Rieker, Patricia and Chloe Bird. 2000. "Sociological explanations of gender differences in mental and physical health." Pp. 98–113 in *Handbook of Medical Sociology,* edited by C. Bird, P. Conrad, and A. Fremont. Upper Saddle River, NJ: Prentice Hall.

Rieker, Patricia and M. Kay Jankowski. 1995. "Sexism and women's psychological status." Pp. 27–50 in *Mental Health, Racism and Sexism,* edited by C. V. Willie, P. P. Rieker, B. Kramer, and B. Brown. Pittsburgh, PA: University of Pittsburgh Press.

Riessman, Catherine. 1983. "Women and medicalization: A new perspective." *Social Policy* 14: 3–18.

Robinson, James C. 1999. *The Corporate Practice of Medicine.* Berkeley, CA: University of California Press.

Roizenblatt, S., Harvey Moldofsky, A.A. Benedito-Silva, and S Tufik. 2001. "Alpha sleep characteristics in fibromyalgia." *Arthritis and Rheumatism* 44: 222–30.

Rosenberg, Charles. 1997. "Introduction framing disease: Illness, society, and history." Pp. xiii–xxvi in *Framing Disease: Studies in Cultural History*, edited by C. Rosenberg and J. Golden. New Brunswick, NJ: Rutgers University Press.

Rosenberg, Charles and Janet Golden, eds. 1997. *Framing Disease: Studies in Cultural History*. New Brunswick, NJ: Rutgers University Press.

Russell, I. Jon, H. Vaeroy, M. Javors, and F. Nyberg. 1992. "Cerebrospinal fluid biogenic amine metabolites in fibromyalgia/fibrositis syndrome and rheumatoid arthritis." *Arthritis and Rheumatism* 35: 550–56.

Ruzek, Sheryl Burt, Virginia Olsen, and Adele Clarke. 1997. *Women's Health: Complexities and Differences*. Columbus, OH: Ohio State University Press.

Sacks, Oliver. 1987. *The Man Who Mistook His Wife for a Hat*. New York: Perennial Library.

Satel, Sally. 2000. *PC, M.D.: How Political Correctness Is Corrupting Medicine*. New York: Basic Books.

Scarry, Elaine. 1985. *The Body in Pain: The Making and Unmaking of the World*. New York: Oxford University Press.

Schutz, Alfred. 1967. "Phenomenology and the Social Sciences." Pp. 118–39 in *Collected Papers, vol. I, The Problem of Social Reality*, edited by M. Natanson. The Hague, Netherlands: M. Nijhoff.

Seccombe, Karen. 1999. *"So You Think I Drive a Cadillac?": Welfare Recipients' Perspectives on the System and Its Reform*. Boston: Allyn and Bacon.

Shorter, Edward. 1992. *From Paralysis to Fatigue: A History of Psychosomatic Illness in the Modern Era*. New York: Free Press.

Showalter, Elaine. 1997. *Hystories: Hysterical Epidemics and Modern Media*. New York: Columbia University Press.

Shryock, Richard Harrison. 1974 [1936]. *The Development of Modern Medicine: An Interpretation of the Social and Scientific Factors Involved*. Madison, WI: University of Wisconsin Press.

Silverstein, Brett and Deborah Perlick. 1995. *The Cost of Competence: Why Inequality Causes Depression, Eating Disorders, and Illness in Women*. New York: Oxford University Press.

Smedley, Brian D., Adrienne Y. Stith, and Alan R. Nelson, eds. 2003. *Unequal Treatment: Confronting Racial and Ethnic Disparities in Health Care*. Washington, DC: National Academies Press.

Smith, Dorothy. 1987. *The Everyday World as Problematic: A Feminist Sociology*. Boston: Northeastern University Press.

Smith-Rosenberg, Carroll. 1985. *Disorderly Conduct: Visions of Gender in Victorian America*. New York: Alfred A. Knopf.

Smyth, Charley, eds. 1985. *Fibrositis and Other Diffuse Musculoskeletal Syndromes*. Philadelphia: Saunders.

Smyth, Charley, Richard Freyberg, and Currier McEwen. 1985. *History of Rheumatology*. Atlanta: Arthritis Foundation.

Smythe, Hugh. 1985. " 'Fibrositis' and other diffuse musculoskeletal syndromes." Pp. 481–89 in *Textbook of Rheumatology, 2nd Edition*, edited by W. N. Kelley, E. D. Harris, S. Ruddy, and C. B. Sledge. Philadelphia: WB Saunders.

Smythe, Hugh. 1972. "Non-articular rheumatism and the fibrositis syndrome." Pp. 874–84 in *Arthritis and Allied Conditions: A Textbook of Rheumatology, 8th Edition*, edited by D. J. McCarthy. Philadelphia: Lea and Febiger.

———. 1979. "Nonarticular rheumatism and psychogenic musculoskeletal syndrome." Pp. 881–91 in *Arthritis and Allied Conditions: A Textbook of Rheumatology*, 9th Edition, edited by D. J. McCarthy. Philadelphia: Lea and Febiger.

———. 1989. "Fibrositis syndrome: A historical perspective." *Journal of Rheumatology, Supplement* 19: 2–6.

Smythe, Hugh and Harvey Moldofsky. 1977. "Two contributions to understanding of the 'fibrositis' syndrome." *Bulletin on the Rheumatic Diseases* 28: 928–31.

Somers, Margaret. 1994. "The narrative construction of identity: A relational and network approach." *Theory and Society* 23: 605–49.

Starlanyl, Devin J. and Mary Ellen Copeland. 1996. *Fibromyalgia and Chronic Myofascial Pain Syndrome: A Survival Manual.* Oakland, CA: New Harbinger Publications.

Starr, Paul. 1982. *The Social Transformation of American Medicine.* New York: Basic Books, Inc.

States of Health. 1996. "Consolidation in the health care market: Good or bad for consumers." *States of Health* 6: 1–8.

Steiner, M., E. Dunn, and L. Born. 2003. "Hormones and mood: From menarche to menopause and beyond." *Journal of Affective Disorders* 74: 67–83.

Stout, A.L., T.A. Grady, J.F. Steege, D.G. Blazer, L.K. George, and M.L. Melville. 1986. "Premenstrual symptoms in black and white community samples." *The American Journal of Psychiatry* 143: 1436–39.

Strauss, Stephen E. 1994. *Chronic Fatigue Syndrome.* New York: Marcel Dekker.

Strazdins, L. and G. Bammer. 2004. "Women, work and musculoskeletal health." *Social Science and Medicine* 58: 997–1005.

Taylor, M.L., D.R. Trotter, and M.E. Csuka. 1995. "The prevalence of sexual abuse in women with fibromyalgia." *Arthritis and Rheumatism* 38: 229–34.

Taylor, Verta. 1995. "Self-labeling and women's mental health: Postpartum illness and the reconstruction of motherhood." *Sociological Focus* 28: 23–47.

Taylor, Verta and Nancy Whittier. 1992. "Collective action in social movement communities: Lesbian feminist mobilization." Pp. 104–129 in *Frontiers in Social Movement Theory*, edited by A. Morris and C. M. Mueller. New Haven, CT: Yale University Press.

Tesh, Syliva Noble. 1988. *Hidden Arguments: Political Ideology and Disease Prevention Policy.* New Brunswick, NJ: Rutgers University Press.

Theriot, Nancy. 1983. "Women's voices in the 19th century medical discourse." *Signs* 19: 1–31.

Turner, Bryan S. 1992. *Regulating Bodies: Essays in Medical Sociology.* London, England: Routledge.

U.S. Census Bureau. 2003. "USA Statistics in Brief: Population and Vital Statistics." Retrieved June 5, 2004 (http://www.census.gov/statab/www/poppart.html).

Umberson, Debra, Meiche D. Chen, James House, Kristin Hopkins, and Ellen Staten. 1996. "The effects of social relationships in psychological well-being:

Are men and women really so different?" *American Sociological Review* 61: 837–57.

Unruh, A.M. 1996. "Gender variations in clinical pain experience." *Pain* 65: 123–67.

Verbrugge, Lois. 1985. "Gender and health: An update on hypotheses and evidence." *Journal of Health and Social Behavior* 26: 156–82.

———. 1990. "Pathways of health and death." Pp. 41–79 in *Women, Health, and Medicine in America: A Historical Handbook*, edited by R.D. Apple. New York: Garland.

Verbrugge, Lois and Deborah Wingard. 1987. "Sex differentials in health and mortality." *Women and Health* 12: 103–45.

Waitzkin, Howard. 1991. *The Politics of Medical Encounters: How Patients and Doctors Deal with Social Problems*. New Haven, CT: Yale University Press.

Waldron, Ingrid. 1995. "Gender and Health-Related Behavior." Pp. 193–208 in *Health Behavior: Emerging Research Perspectives*, edited by D. S. Gochman. New York: Plenum Press.

Walker, E.A., D. Keegan, G. Gardner, M Sullivan, D. Bernstein, and W.J. Katon. 1997. "Psychosocial factors in fibromyalgia compared with rheumatoid arthritis: II. Sexual, physical, and emotional abuse and neglect." *Psychosomatic Medicine* 59: 572–77.

Wallace, Daniel J. and Janice Brock Wallace. 1999. *Making Sense of Fibromyalgia: A Guide for Patients and Their Families*. New York: Oxford University Press.

Wallace, Michelle. 1990. *Black Macho and the Myth of the Superwoman*. London: Verso.

Wallen, J., Howard Waitzkin, and J.D. Stoeckle. 1979. "Physician stereotypes about female health and illness: A study about the informative process during medical interviews." *Women and Health* 4: 135–46.

Ware, Norma C. 1999. "Toward a model of social course in chronic illness: The example of chronic fatigue syndrome." *Culture, Medicine and Psychiatry* 23: 303–31.

Ware, Norma C. and Arthur Kleinman. 1992. "Culture and somatic experience: The social course of illness in neurasthenia and chronic fatigue syndrome." *Psychosomatic Medicine* 54: 546–560.

Warner, John Harley. 1986. *The Therapeutic Perspective*. Cambridge, MA: Harvard University Press.

Waxman, J. and S.M. Zatzkis. 1986. "Fibromyalgia and menopause. Examination of the relationship." *Postgraduate Medicine* 80: 165–67, 170–71.

Weber, Max. 2002 [1904]. *The Protestant Ethic and the Spirit of Capitalism*. Translated by S. Kalberg. Los Angeles: Roxbury Publishing.

Weinblatt, Michael. 2002. "The best of times, the worst of times, rheumatology 2001. ACR presidential address." *Arthritis and Rheumatism* 46: 567–73.

Werner, Anne and Kirsti Malterud. 2003. "It is hard work behaving as a credible patient: Encounters between women with chronic pain and their doctors." *Social Science and Medicine* 57: 1409–19.

Wessley, Simon. 1994. "The history of chronic fatigue syndrome." Pp. 3–44 in *Chronic Fatigue Syndrome*, edited by S. E. Strauss. New York: Marcel Dekker.

White, Evelyn C. 1990. *The Black Women's Health Book*. Seattle: Seal Press.

White, K.P. 2004. "Fibromyalgia: The answer is blowin' in the wind." *Journal of Rheumatology* 31: 636–69.

White, K.P., T. Ostbye, M. Harth, W.R. Neielson, M. Speechley, R. Teasell, and R. Bourne. 2000. "Perspectives on posttraumatic fibromyalgia: A random survey of Canadian general practitioners, orthopedists, physiatrists, and rheumatologists." *Journal of Rheumatology* 27: 790–96.

White, K.P., M. Speechley, M. Harth, and T. Ostbye. 1999. "The London fibromyalgia epidemiology study: The prevalence of fibromyalgia syndrome in London, Ontario." *Journal of Rheumatology* 26: 1570–76.

White, K. P., Nielson W.R., M. Harth, T. Ostbye, and M. Speechley. 2002. "Does the label of "fibromyalgia" alter health status, function, and health service utilization? A prospective, within-group comparison in a community cohort of adults with chronic widespread pain." *Arthritis and Rheumatism* 47: 260–65.

White, K.P. and J. Thompson. 2003. "Fibromyalgia syndrome in an Amish community: A controlled study to determine disease and symptom prevalence." *Journal of Rheumatology* 30: 1835–40.

Williams, Gareth. 1984. "The genesis of chronic illness: Narrative re-construction." *Sociology of Health and Illness* 6: 175–200.

Williamson, Miryam. 1996. *Fibromyalgia: A Comprehensive Approach*. New York: Walker and Company.

Wingard, Deborah. 1997. "Patterns and puzzles: The distribution of health and illness among women in the United States." Pp. 29–50 in *Women's Health: Complexities and Differences*, edited by S. B. Ruzek, V. Olsen, and A. Clarke. Columbus, OH: Ohio State University Press.

Wolfe, Frederick. 1999. "A Reply and Comment by Dr. Frederick Wolfe." Rheuma21st. Retrieved February 15, 2001 (http://www.rheuma21st.com/archives/cutting_edge_fibro_wolfe.html).

———. 2003. "Stop using the American College of Rheumatology criteria in the clinic." *Journal of Rheumatology* 30: 1671–72.

Wolfe, Frederick, J. Anderson, Daniel Harkness, Robert Bennett, Xavier Caro, Don Goldenberg, I. Jon Russell, and Muhammad Yunus. 1997a. "Health status and disease severity in fibromyalgia: Results of a six-center longitudinal study." *Arthritis and Rheumatism* 40: 1571–79.

———. 1997b. "A prospective, longitudinal, multicenter study of service utilization and costs in fibromyalgia." *Arthritis and Rheumatism* 40: 1560–70.

———. 1997c. "Work and disability status of persons with fibromyalgia." *Journal of Rheumatology* 24: 1171–76.

Wolfe, Frederick and Mary Ann Cathey. 1985. "The epidemiology of tender points: A prospective study of 1520 patients." *Journal of Rheumatology* 12: 1164–68.

Wolfe, Frederick, Mary Ann Cathey, S.M. Kleinheksel, S.P. Amos, R.G. Hoffman, D.Y. Young, and Donna Hawley. 1984. "Psychological status in primary fibrositis and fibrositis associated with rheumatoid arthritis." *Journal of Rheumatology* 11: 500–06.

Wolfe, Frederick, Donna Hawley, Mary Ann Cathey, Xavier Caro, and I Jon Russell. 1985. "Fibrositis: Symptom frequency and criteria for diagnosis." *Journal of Rheumatology* 12: 1159–63.

Wolfe, Frederick and Kaleb Michaud. 2004. "Severe rheumatoid arthritis (RA), worse outcomes, comorbid illness, and sociodemographic disadvantage characterize RA patients with fibromyalgia." *Journal of Rheumatology* 31: 695–700.

Wolfe, Frederick, K. Ross, J. Anderson, and I. Jon Russell. 1995a. "Aspects of fibromyalgia in the general population: Sex, pain threshold, and fibromyalgia symptoms." *Journal of Rheumatology* 22: 151–56.

Wolfe, Frederick, K. Ross, J. Anderson, I. Jon Russell, and L. Hebert. 1995b. "The prevalence and characteristics of fibromyalgia in the general population." *Arthritis and Rheumatism* 38: 19–28.

Wolfe, Frederick, Hugh Smythe, Muhammad Yunus, Robert Bennett, Claire Bombardier, Don Goldenberg, Peter Tugwell, Stephen Campbell, Mich Abeles, Patricia Clark, Robert Gatter, Daniel Hamaty, James Lessard, Alan Lichtbrown, Alfonse Masi, Glenn McCain, W. John Reynolds, Thomas Romano, I. Jon Russell, and Robert Sheon. 1990. "The American College of Rheumatology 1990 criteria for the classification of fibromyalgia." *Arthritis and Rheumatism* 33: 160–72.

Wood, Ann Douglass. 1984. "'The fashionable diseases': Women's complaints and their treatment in nineteenth-century America." Pp. 222–38 in *Women and Health,* edited by J. W. Leavitt. Madison, WI: University of Wisconsin Press.

World Health Organization. 1993. *International Statistical Classification of Disease and Related Health Problems,* 10th edition. Geneva: World Health Organization.

Yen, M., R.L. Hough, K. McCabe, A. Lau, and A. Garland. 2004. "Parental beliefs about the causes of child problems: Exploring racial/ethnic patterns." *Journal of the American Academy of Child and Adolescent Psychiatry* 43: 605–12.

Young, Allan. 1995. *The Harmony of Illusions: Inventing Post-Traumatic Stress Disorder.* Princeton, NJ: Princeton University Press.

Young, Iris. 1990. *Throwing Like a Girl and Other Essays in Feminist Philosophy and Social Theory.* Bloomington, IN: Indiana University Press.

Yunus, Muhammad. 1991. "Relationship of clinical features with psychological status of primary fibromyalgia syndrome: Clinical features and association with other functional syndromes." *Arthritis and Rheumatism* 34: 15–21.

———. 1998. "Genetic factors in fibromyalgia syndrome." *Zeitschrift fur Rheumatologie* 57: 61–62.

Yunus, Muhammad, F. Inanici, J.C. Aldag, and R.F. Mangold. 2000. "Fibromyalgia in men: Comparison of clinical features with women." *Journal of Rheumatology* 27: 485–90.

Yunus, Muhammad, Alfonse Masi, John Calabro, Kenneth Miller, and Seth Feigenbaum. 1981. "Primary fibromyalgia (fibrositis): Clinical study of 50 patients with matched normal controls." *Seminars in Arthritis and Rheumatism* 11: 151–171.

Yunus, Muhammad. 2001. "The role of gender in fibromyalgia syndrome." *Current Rheumatology Reports* 3: 128–134.

Yunus, Muhammad, Alfonse Masi, and Jean Aldag. 1989. "A controlled study of primary fibromyalgia syndrome: Clinical features and association with other functional syndromes." *Journal of Rheumatology* 16: 62–71.

Zborowski, Mark. 1969. *People in Pain.* San Francisco: Jossey-Bass.

Index

Waitzkin, Howard, 100, 101
Wallace, Graham, 213
Ware, Norma, 84–85
Watkins, Jennifer, 128
Weber, Max, 8
websites. *See* Internet and websites (FMS)
weight-loss, 99
Weinblatt, Michael, 41–42
welfare, cuts in, 195
Williamson, Miryam. *See Fibromyalgia: A Comprehensive Approach* (Williamson)
wind-up, 31. *See also* pain
Wolfe, Frederick, 23–24, 40, 41, 60
women, 7, 14, 58–59, 60, 105, 196. *See also* feminization; gender; sex; anxiety and, 47; cultural roles of, 47, 48, 53; depression and, 47; discreditation of, 59; health care and, 54; identity of, 135; morbidity and mortality of, 50–51; non-Hispanic white, FMS and, 44–49, 172, 183, 188; pain threshold of, 46; psychosomatic illness and, 63; stress and, 47, 85
women, African American, 53; cultural routinization of pain and, 185–88, 223;

feminists, 186; FMS and, 183; lay medicine and, 187; stress and, 185–86
Women in Pain: Gender and Morbidity in Mexico (Finkler), 56
women patients. *See* patients (FMS)
women's health, 50–54, 198, 212; disparities due to ethnicity, 182–84; gender and, 59, 101; impact of sex and gender on, 49–56; medical literature and, 49; social problems and, 100
women's health movement, 63, 106, 220
women's movement, 62–63, 185
Woodward, Roslyn, 125, 132
work. *See* employment
worker's compensation, 40–41
Worldcat (electronic search tool), 144
World Health Organization (WHO), 26, 153

x-rays, 4, 95.

yeast infections, FMS and, 66, 181
Yunus, Muhammad, 23–24, 214

Zborowski, Mark, 184

Kristin K. Barker is Assistant Professor of Sociology at Oregon State University.